Endc

MW00987279

T his book is a remarkab psychological skills ai healing principles of trauma psychology with holistic psychiatry. Dr. Whitfield explains in some detail how the reader can use practical and proven non-drug techniques and recovery aids to handle their psychological, emotional and behavioral symptoms. Caution: This book contains an indictment of the psychiatric drug industry and an enlightening exposure of their dogma for the people who are taking these brain disabling drugs and those who care for them.

—Peter R. Breggin, MD, psychiatrist
Author of *Medication Madness*, Ithaca, NY

I have known Charles Whitfield for 20 years and believe that this is the most telling and powerful of his several books on mental health and recovery. As a longtime psychology professor and clinician I am impressed with how clearly and concisely he describes what causes the emotional, behavioral and relationship pain for those labeled as "mentally ill" and then what works best to heal their problems. He also tells the truth about how and why psychiatric drugs don't work well and too often make people worse. Highly recommended.

—Randy Noblitt, PhD, Professor of
Clinical Psychology,
The California School of Professional Psychology
Author of reference [118]

On the Cover

The man standing with his back to us looking out at the clear and wondrous landscape represents the promise and actuality of healing and recovery from the bothersome and painful effects of repeated hurts, losses and traumas that have been misdiagnosed as though they were mental illness and mistreated—usually with drugs that don't work well or make many people worse. He has risen above and from his previously painful life of confusion and despair as shown at the lower left of the cover art and his frustration from trying to find relief from it with numerous prescribed psychiatric drugs unsuccessfully, as shown at the lower right.

Throughout this book I describe the clear and wondrous landscape of recovery and healing that he is now seeing. But it is not an easy journey. This landscape includes finding and naming the original traumas we experienced and those traumas we are experiencing now from others labeling us as "mentally ill" or "disordered," giving and sometimes forcing toxic drugs on us and helping professionals who don't listen to us and don't guide us in the right direction to heal. As you read, please look carefully at the several tables and charts in the Appendix.

The original painting without the lower imagery was by Caspar David Fredrich, a German Romance painter of the 19th century. This image was found to be in the public domain. Friedrich came of age during a period when across Europe a growing disillusionment with materialistic society was giving rise to a new appreciation of spirituality. Friedrich said,

"The artist should paint not only what he sees before him, but also what he sees within him."

Charles L. Whitfield, M.D.

NOT CRAZY
YOU MAY NOT BE MENTALLY ILL

MISDIAGNOSED AND MISTREATED WITH DRUGS
THAT DON'T WORK WELL
OR MAKE YOU WORSE

IMPORTANT INFORMATION WITHHELD FROM YOU
BY THE DRUG INDUSTRY, PSYCHIATRY,
GOVERNMENT, AND OTHERS

by

CHARLES L. WHITFIELD, MD

Best-selling Author of
Healing the Child Within
and the two-volume pair,

The Truth About Depression
and
The Truth About Mental Illness

ᄳᄒP
muse house press

MUSE HOUSE PRESS

ISBN: 978-1-935827-02-3

Charles L. Whitfield, M.D.

Acknowledgements

Thanks to my wife Barbara Whitfield for assisting me with typing and her excellent feedback while drafting this book.

Thanks to Donald Brennan for his usual excellent layout and graphics work on this book.

Thanks to my countless patients over the decades who have given me the opportunity to learn from them — much of which is in this book.

Thanks to Peter Breggin MD for his exemplary and clear work and encouragement, much of which is reflected throughout this book.

Thanks to J Douglas Bremner MD for his contributions to the trauma psychology and psychiatry literature, reflected throughout this book.

Thanks to the Leadership Council on Child Abuse and Interpersonal Violence board members for their ongoing contributions, many of which are reflected throughout this book.

And to all my other colleagues in the Trauma Field for their bravery in naming the truth of what they see in their patients, clients and countless research subjects, also reflected throughout this book .

Thanks to Alan Gaby MD who once was my student and later taught me about supplements and how they work.

I would like to thank Lindsay Jenkins at Lightning Source for her patience and gracious help in publishing this book whose time has come.

Finally to the legal psychiatric drug industry, without which I would not have needed to write this book.

Dedication

I dedicate this book to all people who read it with an open mind and with empathy and not preconceived beliefs.*

I dedicate this book to my countless patients over the decades who have given me the opportunity to learn from them—much of which is incorporated in this book.

I dedicate this book to all trauma survivors who have been misdiagnosed and mistreated.

I dedicate this book to all clinicians who work to assist these trauma survivors.

I dedicate this book to my colleagues in medicine and psychiatry in hopes that they will take a careful trauma history and help those patients who want to taper off of psychiatric drugs and especially for those who are made worse by them.

And finally, to the psychiatric drug industry (aka BigPharma) without which I would not have needed to write this book.

* I base this on a classic quote from the Alcoholics Anonymous "*Big Book.*"

"*There is a principle which is a bar against all information, which is proof against all arguments, and which cannot fail to keep a man in everlasting ignorance. That principle is* **contempt prior to investigation**."

—Herbert Spencer

(Quoted in the AA Big Book's appendices), as well as from the work of Peter Breggin, Pim van Lommel, Neal Grossman, many others and ours in *The Power of Humility*.

Table of Contents

Introduction

Countless people across the USA and world are being misdiagnosed and mistreated for "mental illness" that they do not have. The problem is that only a few helping professionals are pointing this out. [21,108,109,132,141.142,153,173,174,185] There are too few whistle blowers.

After seeing many of my patients for years who had been mislabeled and mistreated, I have now written this book to tell you what I have observed and what the truth may be for them—and possibly for you or someone who you may know. I have written it to summarize how you and they can finally begin to heal and recover without psychiatric drugs. This summary includes finding and naming the original traumas we experienced and those traumas we are experiencing now from toxic drugs and clinicians who don't listen to us and don't guide us in the right direction to heal. I describe how to accomplish these do-able tasks in this book.

Some readers will be skeptical about what I say. They may believe that they have a reasonable explanation for their problems and pain. They are convinced that they are "mentally ill." For some their symptoms may have been helped for a time by their taking a psychiatric drug, such as an antidepressant, an antipsychotic, a "mood stabilizer" or some other drug.

Others may have believed that they might have a mental illness because they have been told by someone else—a clinician, family member or friend or by reading a book or article. But do they or you have to believe that? Is there a better way out?

Whatever your situation, persuasion or preference, you may consider reading what I have observed and learned about mental illness, healing and recovery from countless of my patients and the scientific literature over the past 3-plus decades.

1   Why You May NOT Be Mentally Ill

WAYS OUT OF THE PAINFUL EFFECTS OF WRONG DIAGNOSIS AND WRONG TREATMENT

Have you—or someone you know or care about—been diagnosed with "mental illness" such as depression, bipolar disorder, anxiety disorder, ADHD, or the like? If so how were you treated by your health professionals? Did their treatment help you? Or did it help the people you know? Did they prescribe drugs? Did the treatment make you worse? Did they offer any other recovery aids? Or perhaps you are not sure?

I ask these same questions of clinicians who may be reading this book. Have you treated or assisted people with any of these problems? Have you noticed that diagnostic labels and drugs didn't work as well as they should to help them heal? Did any of the treatments make any of them worse?

There is increasing evidence that the current medical and mental health treatment systems are not helping most of those we would like them to help. [21,25,74,108,109,132,141,142,153,173,174,185]   In my over 30 years assisting countless people with a variety of mental, emotional, behavioral and relationship problems, I have come to realize that many of them have been misdiagnosed and mistreated. In fact, *most* of them who were previously diagnosed with a "mental illness" were not mentally ill. Instead, most were suffering from one or more of the effects of repeated childhood and later abuse, trauma and neglect. Their mental, emotional, behavioral, and relationship problems were the neuro-developmental and patho-physiological results of their growing up being repeatedly abused, neglected and otherwise traumatized.

FACTORS IN MISDIAGNOSIS AND MISTREATMENT

I have seen at least nine causes or reasons why people may be misdiagnosed and mistreated for symptoms of "mental illness," which I summarize in Table 1 and begin to discuss below and then describe throughout this book.

1 POST-TRAUMATIC STRESS DISORDER (PTSD)

Instead of their being "mentally ill," with any of the above mental illness or disorder labels, I found that most of my patients had post-traumatic stress disorder (PTSD). [32,71,173,174] Some of them had a more advanced form of PTSD, which is called complex PTSD (see page 51). [32,43,71] Sure, on the surface most had the *symptoms* of various mental illnesses. But underneath was usually PTSD or the toxic effects of psychiatric drugs, or both.

PTSD is not a mental illness or disorder. Rather, it is a normal reaction to an abnormal, i.e., traumatic experience. Others [27,32,34,43,56,57,59,71,92,137,157,182] and I [173,174] have found that underlying whatever surface problem or "mental disorder" a person may at first appear to have, there will often be PTSD. We commonly see people with PTSD to have an exaggeration of one or more of its features, such as anxiety (a modern code word for fear), depression (a common code word for stuck grief or numbness), and aggressive or violent behavior (common code words for unresolved anger or resentment).

Among those people with the more advanced or complex PTSD, we may see problems with more severe dissociation (separation from emotional pain), such as multiple personality (also called dissociative identity disorder), or a deeper dissociation called a psychosis (schizophrenia and the like – which are usually extreme disorders of fear and shame).

If the PTSD is not recognized and diagnosed, given the unsuccessful state of our mental health care delivery system today (look at your own or others' lives and experiences), it is likely that most trauma survivors will be mislabeled and thereby be mistreated. Currently that mistreatment is by prescribing for them a psychiatric drug that will likely be toxic to their mental, emotional, behavioral, physical and spiritual well-being, which I describe throughout this book. Instead of helping the person with

Table 1.1. Why You May NOT be Mentally Ill and Ways Out of Emotional & Behavioral Pain

Why You *May NOT* Be Mentally Ill...	Ways Out of Emotional & Behavioral Pain
You may : 1. – be **misdiagnosed**, and instead, have **PTSD** (or other **trauma effects**)	→Realize that PTSD & other trauma effects (e.g., depression, anxiety, etc)[1] are caused most often by repeated traumas. →Begin a stage-oriented recovery program.
2. - be **grieving** a loss, hurt or trauma	→Identify & name the loss, hurt, or trauma. →Learn the process of grieving & let yourself feel your feelings & grieve over time as long as it may take. [2]
3. - be involved in one or more **toxic relationships**	→Identify & name the relationships as hurtful, abusive or toxic. Set healthy boundaries with them [3], [4]

---

[1] See e.g. *The Truth About Depression* 2003 & *The Truth About Mental Illness* 2004
[2] See e.g. *Healing the Child Within* or *A Gift to Myself*
[3] See *Boundaries and Relationships*
[4] See *Codependence: Healing the Human Condition*

**Table 1.1 Why You May NOT be Mentally Ill and
Ways Out of Emotional & Behavioral Pain**... *continued*

Why You *May NOT* Be Mentally Ill...	*Ways Out of Emotional & Behavioral Pain*
You may: 4) - have **toxic drug effects** or withdrawal symptoms	→Identify & name the drug & that your symptoms are due to its effects or to its withdrawal [1]
5) - be **forced** (by court or the like) **to take** toxic **drugs** or **ECT**	→Locate & see a clinician with expertise in forced drugging. →See also: www.mindfreedom.org
6) - be an abused, neglected,"hurried," or mis-educated child or person	→Realize that e.g., ADHD, bipolar disorder, etc. are far over- and mis-diagnosed & mis-treated in adults & kids [1]
7) - have an active physical illness or addiction	→Know that stress & trauma are major causes of these & that active addiction is a common generator of "MI" symptoms.
8) - have a combination of the above	→Begin a stage-oriented recovery program. [2]
9) - have a **clinician** who **doesn't have skills** in helping with the above	→Find & see a clinician with expertise in trauma recovery. →Stop calling yourself "Mentally Ill."

their presenting symptoms or problems, these drugs may instead, over time, make them worse.

2 GRIEVING

Instead of being "mentally ill," you—or the person you know—may be grieving a loss, hurt or trauma. In my years of clinical practice I have seen many people who had been misdiagnosed with "depression" or another "mental illness" who were actually sad or distressed because they had experienced a major loss, hurt or trauma. They were in the active process of grieving or they were in a less active or "stuck" state of acute or chronic grief. And usually someone had prescribed one or more psychoactive drugs, which had not helped their emotional pain and often made them worse.

An example:

Bill was a 45-year-old man who had been treated with 3 different antidepressant drugs for "depression" for the past 2 years. He came to me for a second opinion, since his sadness, low energy, and quality of life were now worse than when he started the drugs. He had gained 40 pounds and felt mostly numb. On taking a more detailed history, which he said his prescribing physicians had not done, he had been undergoing a painful separation and divorce during these two years when he was diagnosed as being "depressed." Instead of having a distinct disorder that his prior physicians had labeled as "depression," I suggested that he actually might be grieving the loss of a marriage of many years, with all its hopes, dreams and vows now lost. I suggested that he might not be mentally ill, and over the course of the next year he was able to taper the dose of his antidepressant and begin to grieve his hurts and losses, using psychotherapy and self-help group meetings and literature, plus an exercise program.

This scenario may be the case for many people in such a situation. A problem is that today many if not most psychiatrists and other physicians are not adequately trained or oriented to identify and treat acute and chronic grief. And some non-physician clinicians may have known of his separation and divorce but did not caution him about the toxic effects of the antidepressant drugs.

3   TOXIC RELATIONSHIPS

Another common reason why you may not be mentally ill is that you – or someone you know – might be involved in a toxic relationship. Your interactions with that toxic person or persons may be so stressful and even distressing that *as a result* you are experiencing painful feelings or behaving in dysfunctional ways or doing things that you may not want to do.

The way out of your pain may *not* be to label yourself as being "mentally ill" or to accept such a label from anyone else. Your way out may *not* be to take a drug. Being in the toxic relationship may likely be the cause of your distress.

The way out is first to identify and name the relationship as hurtful, abusive or toxic. Then you can set healthy boundaries and limits with them regarding their hurtful or abusive behavior (for other ways out, also consider looking at my book *Boundaries and Relationships*).

Handling toxic relationships can also seem daunting, but I offer three recovery aids below that you can consider doing to deal with toxic relationships.

1) Attend Twelve Step meetings such as Al-Anon where you can learn how to detach from abusive people), Co-dependents Anonymous (CoDA, where you can learn how you may be a part of the toxic relationship problem);

2) Use psychotherapy or counseling to work through your associated issues; and,

6

3) Use bibliotherapy (read helpful books, such as Al-Anon, ACA (Adult-Children Anonymous) or CoDA literature and the like (*Boundaries and Relationships*).

4 TOXIC DRUG EFFECTS

Another reason why you may not be mentally ill is that the drug(s) you are taking for your assumed "mental disorder" may instead be a major part of the problem. The drug or drugs may be causing or significantly aggravating your mental, emotional, behavioral and relationship problems. A psychiatric drug may be toxic due to its *direct* effects, such as over-sedation or over-stimulation, or to *indirect* effects, such as drug withdrawal. The best way to handle such a problem is to identify and *name* the drug's specific *toxicity* and determine that your symptoms are due to these effects, which may also include drug withdrawal. I describe these problems and how to recognize and handle them in Chapters 7, 8, 9 and 12, and in Table A.1-6 in the Appendix (p 199).

Caution: Don't suddenly stop taking a psychiatric drug unless you are advised to do so by a health professional. For example, if you have **akathisia** (a very emotionally and often physically painful inner restlessness and irritability that usually masks as "mental illness"—even to clinicians who you may consult) during the early weeks of starting an antidepressant or antipsychotic drug, it is usually advisable to stop the drug now. A problem is that akathisia can come on during drug withdrawal as well, for which you may need to taper the drug if you had taken it long term (here it would be best to consult an expert in drug toxicity).

5 FORCED DRUGGING

Forcing people to take psychiatric drugs or to have electro convulsive shock treatment (ECT) is an unfortunate effect of the interplay between our legal and psychiatric systems. But it is usually a toxic short cut to resolving behavior problems. I address forced drugging in Chapter 10 on page 114.

6 TRAUMA HISTORY
(abused, neglected, "hurried," or mis-educated)

Diagnosis and Misdiagnosis: People with a history of repeated childhood and/or later abuse or neglect are at high risk for being diagnosed or misdiagnosed with one or more mental disorders. Up until 2003 and 4, when I published my two books *The Truth about Depression* and *The Truth about Mental Illness*, the scientific data were *strong* (for most mental illness) to *overwhelming* (for depression and addictions) that a significant trauma history is common among people with symptoms of mental illness, as summarized in Table 1.2. From 2004 until now, these same results continue to be seen, compiled and published (e.g., ACE study results ongoing, [57] John Read's publications, [128] and more).

This table has a lot of information. Look especially at the far left and far right columns which show how many studies document the links to having a history of repeated trauma. (Refer to my books *The Truth about Depression* and *The Truth about Mental Illness* for details.)

The data are clear from the over 350 peer reviewed published studies that compile the table. Mental, emotional, behavioral pain and disrupted relationships—the prime symptoms of mental disorders —are commonly due to having experienced repeated trauma. But our "mental health" system is not aware and skilled enough to handle these symptoms and behaviors as being trauma effects.

Most clinicians are not sufficiently trained to diagnose and treat them in this more effective way. Thus, most people with these symptoms and problems get misdiagnosed as having one or more "mental disorders," and then mistreated with psychiatric drugs that are themselves toxic to our mind and body.

Treatment and Mistreatment: Almost every trauma survivor who comes to me for assistance had been prescribed, either voluntarily or by force, at least one toxic drug. Most had been given several, and some had a history of having taken from 10 to 20 or more of these drugs over time with little or most often no success. One example of how often trauma survivors get treated or mistreated with psych drugs is found in a recent prospective study of adults in the San Diego, California area from 1997 to 2004. Of these 15,033 people, 5,480 of them said that they had *no history* of childhood trauma (called Adverse Childhood Experiences or "ACEs" in this study). The remainder – 9,553 people – reported having had a *history of* one or more *repeated childhood traumas.* In every single one of these 8 separate-year periods surveyed before the study began the researchers found an increased and graded relationship between having a trauma history and later being prescribed psychiatric drugs. This graded relationship occurred in an increasing or stair-step pattern wherein the more trauma history these 9,553 people experienced, the more psych drugs they received, [7,57] as shown in Figures 1.1 and 1.2 below.

This is a remarkable study. It is the first to show a link between trauma and subsequent psychiatric drug use. It shows how the more repeated trauma a person experiences, the more likely they are to be prescribed—either forced or unforced—toxic psychiatric drugs. This likelihood of being prescribed psych drugs was here increased by a *highly significant* factor of from 2 to 17 times versus those people with no childhood trauma histories. [57] Based on these highly significant results on such a large sample of the general population, it is likely that countless other trauma survivors are today being given toxic psychiatric drugs for "mental illness" that they do not have—which I describe in detail throughout this book.

Table 1.2 Number of Studies that Document a Link Between Childhood Trauma & Mental Illness [174]

Clinical Area	Clinical	Community	Prospective	Index/Meta-Analys/LitRev	Strength of Data/Total #
Depression	96	70	22	21/2*	Overwhelming/ 327 (see p. 255)
Suicidality		22 (both)		7	Strong/29
Alcohol/Drug Probs (SA/CD)		90	21	42 Index, 11 M-A/LitRev	Powerful/ 153
Eating Disorders		58	7	43 index 7 Lit	Very Strong/ 108
PTSD	54	21	10	0/6	Strong/85
Anxiety Disorder	35	38	12	15/2	Very Strong/ 100
Personality Disorders		35	5	36/1	Very Strong/ 76
Psychosis		67	4 (& 2 strong family studies)	37 index 8 lit reviews	Very strong/ 110
ADHD		58	15	4/3	Strong/77
Aggression & Violence		40	16	10	Strong/66
Low Self-Esteem	17	10	4	Only 1 of 31 didn't find it	Strong/31
Dissociative Disorders	30	16	3	11/2	Strong/57
Nicotine		10	1		Suggestive to Firm/11
Somatization		38	11	16	Strong/65
Revictimization		38	1	4	Firm to Strong/ 38 (see p. 208)

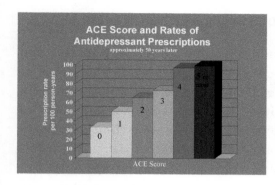

Figure1.1
Antidepressants*

*Similar results were found for "mood stabilizers," which is a marketing term for expensive and toxic anti-convulsants *and* were found for antipsychotics. [57]

As numerous psychiatrists and others have shown, these are not benign chemicals. For a sizeable percentage of people who take them, they are potent, stressing and distressing. Their effects are commonly so distressing over time that they become traumatic to the user in their effects alone, thereby heaping more trauma upon those already trying to heal from the painful and disabling effects of repeated childhood and later traumas as I show in Chapter 7.

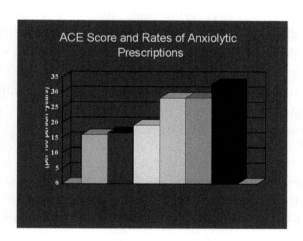

Figure 1.2 Anti-anxiety drugs (from Felitti & Anda 2010 [57])

11

7   An Active Addiction or Physical Illness

A basic principle in addiction medicine, psychiatry and psychology is that active alcohol or drug *addiction can mimic or simulate almost every mental illness*, and at times some physical illnesses. Active addiction itself is also a common generator of most of the symptoms of mental illness. The wise clinician usually wants their patient to be off of alcohol and/or drugs for a few weeks and preferably months before diagnosing them with a mental illness—at which time the person's original symptoms are often much improved or gone. At that point, no additional diagnoses are appropriate for a large percentage of such people.

Thus, if one has an addiction to alcohol or other drugs, or at times to gambling or the like, they may not otherwise be mentally ill.

8   An Unaware or Unskilled Clinician

Most physicians, including psychiatrists, are not sufficiently trained in recognizing the above possible causal factors that can and commonly do cause symptoms and signs of mental illness. Over the past 25 years, medical schools, residency training programs and especially continuing medical education events have gradually been influenced and taken over by the legal drug industry. Medicine and psychiatry have lost their independence from the undue influence of Big Pharma in all of its guises and disguises. (see Figure 11.1 on page 133).

Even the *DSM* (*Diagnostic and Statistical Manual of Mental Disorders*—the diagnostic "bible" of psychiatry) is in large part tainted by the legal drug industry's influence. For example, most of the DSM's committee members who write the description and diagnostic criteria for each mental disorder receive a significant amount of their income from one and usually several drug companies. [1,2,87,132,162,173,174,185] This kind of pay-off is also rampant in other areas of medicine and psychiatry, from medical researchers to medical school faculty to journal article authors to Food and Drug Administration committee members to professional groups such as the American Psychiatric Association. Most medical and psychiatric journals depend on drug advertising to stay active, and congress and the White House are lobbied strongly and regularly by Big Pharma and other drug promoters. People of all ages are inundated by TV drug advertisements, which were illegal until 1981 when Big Pharma bought with lobby money the approval by congress for them to hawk their toxic wares.

The health insurance industry is also partially to blame. While their CEOs each earn multi-millions in income, they limit the payment for each of your personal doctor visits and your total number of visits, forcing medical and psychiatric physicians to spend a usually inadequate and short amount of time per patient.

An old saying goes "If the only tool you have is a hammer, everything you see looks like a nail." This translates – If all you know is *how to label* (required by the health insurance industry) someone *with a mental disorder* and *prescribe drugs*, you will tend not to see or do much else for your patients or clients.

Some other clinicians are often similarly involved in misdiagnosing and mistreating people. Some get caught in the same spiders web of BigPharma and BigInsurance. I have also observed several of my colleagues, including social workers, counselors, psych nurses, and an occasional psychologist who themselves were on one or more psych drugs, commonly for their "depression" or "bipolar" condition. Over time I got to know most of them fairly well, and every one of them had a history of repeated childhood trauma. Unfortunately, for one reason or another, they encouraged their own clients to do what they had done.

The way out of the original emotional, behavioral and physical pain, and out of the drug-induced pain is to find and see a clinician with expertise in assisting with trauma recovery. Develop your own personal recovery plan. [175] And stop calling yourself "mentally ill."

9   A COMBINATION OF THE ABOVE

In my experience, most of the people who I have seen in my practice have a combination of these above factors that help explain why you—or someone you know—may actually not be mentally ill. It usually takes time to consider each of these possibilities and to sort them out, and then to begin the hard and long work of healing and recovery, which I have described in my other books in some detail and which I will summarize and update in the following chapters. Most physicians, including most psychiatrists today do not know, understand or believe what I describe throughout this book.

So before you jump into the middle of such a recovery program, it may be helpful to know about some more factors and potential road blocks to your reaching success. I will address these in the next chapter.

2   Genesis — How Did this Happen?

GENESIS AND DEVELOPMENT

For those who may have grown up in—or still be living in—a dysfunctional, unhealthy or painful family, relationship or world, it can be useful to explore how we have arrived here. As a child we may have been repeatedly mistreated, abused or neglected. To survive, our Real Self, True Self (Child Within) went into hiding (dissociated, separated) deep within the unconscious part of our psyche [167,181]. To try to run our life, our false self (ego) took over. But it was not able to do the job. Over time, we may have felt more and more emotional pain, distressed, and at times even "crazy."

Others—our parents or parent figures—who likely, at least in part, caused our mental and our emotional pain back then—may today use a diagnosis or label of some kind of "mental illness" to help keep us dysfunctional and to control us further. These others still may project their own unfinished business onto us. Unaware of how to get out of this situation, and to continue to survive, we continue to take this abuse into our conscious and unconscious awareness ("unhealthy introjects," in psychological terms), including the idea, theory or claim that we are "mentally ill."

The effects of all of the above—our original trauma plus our ongoing traumas—may look or feel like "mental illness." The kind(s) of "mental disorder" that surface for any person usually depend on the type and intensity of the abuse, the developmental age when they were abused, what others—especially parents—model or teach, and other factors.

What results from a lifetime of repeated trauma may vary from person to person. If looked for and carefully considered, many people will find that they have PTSD or complex PTSD. They also may develop psychological patterns and lifestyles that help lessen their emotional pain temporarily. Some will surface as having one or more addictions. Others will have "depression," various "anxiety disorders," "dissociative disorders," "personality disorders," "ADHD" or "ADD," "bipolar disorder," or a "psychosis"— or a *combination* of these (called "dual disorders" or "co-morbidity" in the psychiatry, psychology and counseling trades, although most of these diagnoses are due to repeated trauma).

These may appear to be separate and distinct entities, disorders or illnesses. But as over 400 independent researchers world-wide have shown scientifically, underlying and at the base of every one of these is a history of repeated childhood and later trauma (Table 1.2 on page 10 above). These facts remain true in spite of their denial by most of medicine, psychiatry, much of psychology, and related helping professions, groups, organizations and authorities—both governmental and independent. [173, 174]

Today, most people who are given these "diagnoses" or labels will then automatically be given toxic psych drugs which usually do not work well, if at all, and often make them worse. Some will be given electro convulsive treatment. And some will be *forced* to take these.

Most will not be asked about a trauma history or offered treatment aids other than drugs. A problem is that in this incomplete process most people are thereby misdiagnosed and mistreated, which often add yet another perhaps subtle but real trauma to their painful experiences of abuse and neglect.

Some readers may wonder or ask "what about the genetic idea or abnormal brain chemistry explanation of the cause of mental illness?" The fact is that the genetic transmission belief is only a now popular *theory* that has never been definitively proven, as research psychologist Jay Joseph and others clearly describe. The

16

methodology of the research that has tried to prove this genetic theory is weak at best and totally erroneous at worst. [82,132,173,174] Because some mental, emotional, and behavior problems run in families does not prove the genetic theory, since child abuse and neglect also runs in families. And the direct face to face examination of family members in *essentially all genetic research rarely* goes back even one full generation. Most of the information on the parents and grandparents in these studies comes from only the present adult generation, and thus is at best hearsay and at worst unreliable.

The same principle applies to the abnormal brain chemistry *theory* of the cause of mental illness, as others have documented [25,109,161,162,173,174,195] which I summarize in Table A 9 on page 216 in the Appendix. There is **no available reliable** or **definitive diagnostic laboratory**, **blood**, **urine**, or any other body fluid or tissue test **for any** of the **common mental illnesses**.

The current diagnosis of mental illness is based on *DSM* diagnostic criteria (simply symptoms and observable signs that anyone can ask about or look for) that are **voted on** by the *simple consensus* of mostly academic psychiatrists and a small few people from other professions. **Nearly all** of these receive a significant percentage of their **income from the drug industry**, which is clearly a conflict of interest. [87,132,162,173,174,185,196,200]

In limited ways such diagnostic criteria are better than having none at all. The *DSM*'s main *advantages* are its usefulness 1) for health insurance reimbursement documentation, 2) for research purposes, and clinically 3) for adding to the process and structure of making an early treatment plan. It's *dis*advantages are that it 1) is based more on theory than scientific fact, it 2) labels people with a stigma that can interfere with their personal freedom, opportunity and dignity, and 3) in the last 25-plus years it has become contaminated by both a subtle and overt invasion by the drug industry. [42,87,185,196] While it may have some potential as a way to begin to make sense of human suffering and behavior, it remains oversimplified, and except for including PTSD as a bona fide condition, it tends to ignore having a trauma history in its differential diagnosis sections.

The idea of "mental illness" is no more than a theory, hypothesis, or a construct. As mentioned above, there is no firm, convincing or definitive proof for its two most claimed causes: genetic transmission and abnormal brain chemistry. Its main treatments—drugs and ECT—damage the brain and body and tend not to work well. [108,109,132,141.142,153,173,174,185] By contrast, many people often slowly get better when their symptoms are reframed as trauma effects and they work a *full trauma-based recovery* program *with patience* and *persistence.* [92,164,165,173,174,181]

So how did this come about? Here is a summary that I describe in more detail in the next 2 chapters.

- Others who caused or aggravated the effects/symptoms may use the diagnosis of "mental illness" to help keep me dysfunctional.

- These others project(ed) *their own* unfinished business onto me.

- Then I take this abuse into my unconscious and conscious awareness (unhealthy introjects), [67,93,181] including that I am "mentally ill."

- In the process, to survive the pain (hurt, shame, guilt, fear), my child within (real self) went into hiding.

- My false self (ego) was left to run my life, though it was incapable of doing so.

- The effect(s) of all this, plus ongoing hurts, losses and traumas, may look or feel like "mental illness," when they are not.

- The kind(s) of "mental illness" that surface usually depend on the type and intensity of the abuse, the developmental age abused, what others (esp. parents) model or teach, and other factors.

Instead of "mental illness," many of us will actually have PTSD or complex PTSD, with or without the following:

- Some will surface as addiction(s), others as "depression," various "anxiety disorders," "dissociative disorders," "personality disorders," "ADHD or ADD," "bipolar disorder," or a psychosis --or a combination of these.

- Many with these assumed "diagnoses" will be given toxic psychiatric drugs and/or ECT (electro convulsive treatment) which often do not work and make them worse. [25,26,179]

- Some will be *forced* to take the drugs and/or ECT.

- Most will **not** be asked about a trauma history or offered more recovery methods than drugs.

BE CAREFUL — 8 CAUTIONS

Before you start to make any changes in your life or your current treatment aids, and before you talk to *anyone* in your family of origin or *any* authority figure or clinician about any of your developing ideas or insights about why you may not be mentally ill, consider the following 8 cautions. Others and I have found these principles to remain valid over time.

1) Don't stop taking any psych drug suddenly or without medical supervision (see Chapter 12).

2) If you do decide to stop, do so slowly and with knowledgeable and expert medical supervision. It usually takes weeks at best, but usually months, and sometimes a year or more to fully withdraw and detox from many of these drugs. Use a nutritional program to aid an easier withdrawal process.

3) If you have PTSD, unless you begin and maintain a full recovery program for trauma effects, be careful of ignoring your current treatment plan.

4) Be careful who you talk to about your insights of not being "mentally ill." A quote from author Joseph Campbell may help here: "The difference between a psychotic and a mystic (a spiritually evolved person) is that the mystic knows who not to talk to (about their psycho-spiritual insights)."

5) Be prepared that family, friends, and many clinicians will likely react negatively if you try to share your insights with them.

6) Know that just because you may now have this insight or reframe, many of your symptoms will likely not automatically go away.

7) You will likely still need the assistance of actively participating in an appropriate full recovery program.

8) What brought you to your current problems-in-living may take a long time to discover, name and work through.

With these eight principles and cautions in mind, I have found the following flow chart (also called a decision tree or algorithm) to be useful when contemplating what to do next. Take your time. There is usually *no rush to jump into a sudden change* prematurely.

Has a helping professional given me a diagnosis of any mental disorder or illness?

Do I wonder if I may be mentally ill?

Read over the words in each box in the chart and consider where you may likely be right now and where you could be later.

Study it carefully.

If you have any questions, read as much of the rest of this book as you have the time and interest to do. If you have any urgent mental, emotional or behavioral needs, immediately contact and see a mental health professional, preferably a licensed psychologist, licensed clinical social worker or a licensed counselor.

If they try to push you to take psychiatric drugs, be careful. You might want to get a second or third opinion. Most physicians and nearly all psychiatrists will try to push psych drugs on you. Of course, don't try to stop taking them without expert clinical assistance. Read Chapter 12 on stopping drugs first.

A short cut to what further actions you can consider begins on page 170 on recovery, but I recommend being as patient as you can while reading the other chapters in between before beginning Chapter 14. Of course, it always is up to you.

Figure 2.1. Flow Chart on decision making about my symptoms & potential actions to help me heal

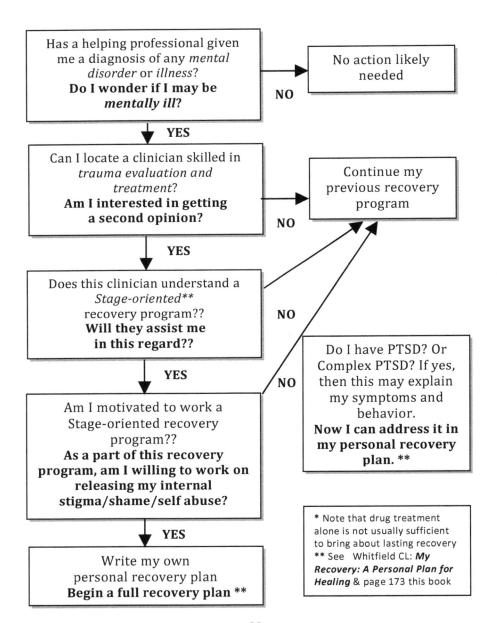

3   The Process of Trauma

Trauma is any event that significantly harms the body, self or spirit. It covers a broad range of hurtful experiences including traumas that involve the physical, sexual, mental or emotional realms of our being. The main kinds of childhood trauma include sexual abuse (CSA), physical abuse (CPA), and psychological or emotional abuse. Child emotional and physical neglect are also traumatic, as is *witnessing* verbal or physical violence, especially within the family, and having a mentally ill household member. [56,57] Loss of a parent or parent figure through separation, divorce or death is also traumatic.

These traumas may occur under different guises that may go unrecognized by the victim, perpetrator and observer as being traumatic, as summarized in Figure 3.1. on the next page.

Childhood and other trauma experiences are complex. Clinical and research psychologist William Friedrich said, "To simply place a broad label on a child as sexually abused may allow for a simple categorization, but it obscures the heterogeneity [variation and diversity], severity, and co-occurrence of maltreatment experiences." [59] Each kind of abuse usually occurs in combination with one or more of the others, with psychological/emotional abuse being the most common and nearly always present in the background of the other three main trauma types, as shown in Figure 3.2 on page 25.

There are several avenues through which we can explore the genesis and dynamics of trauma and its effects. I summarize how this usually happens in the following section on the process of wounding. If it appears to be ponderous, please bear with me. Or skip to another section and return later, as it is important to understand how repeated childhood trauma hurts us.

Figure 3.1. Childhood Trauma v Healthy Parenting [173]

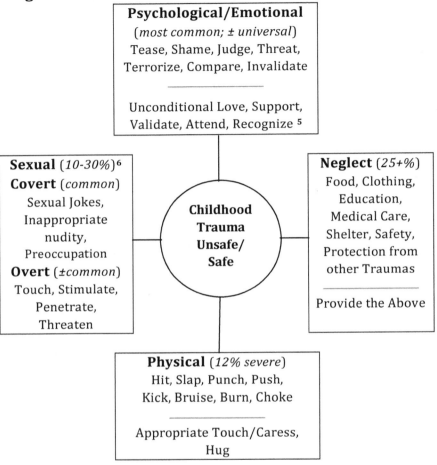

---

[5] Healthy parenting descriptors are shown below the line in 3 boxes as appropriate.

[6] These % figures are estimates of the incidence & prevalence of these types of childhood trauma, based on data from the literature. Paradoxically, statistics based on reports of *child protective services* may show the opposite of the actual occurrence of trauma. These figures are (actual occurrence/CPS reports), *neglect* (25+/50+ %), *physical* (12%/18%), *sexual* (10-30%/9%), *emotional* (90%/4%). Most *published clinical and research* data are on (in order of most common study data): sexual, physical, these two combined, psychological and very little on neglect. [173]

Charles L. Whitfield, M.D.

Figure 3.2. Venn Diagram of the Spectrum of Childhood Trauma [7]

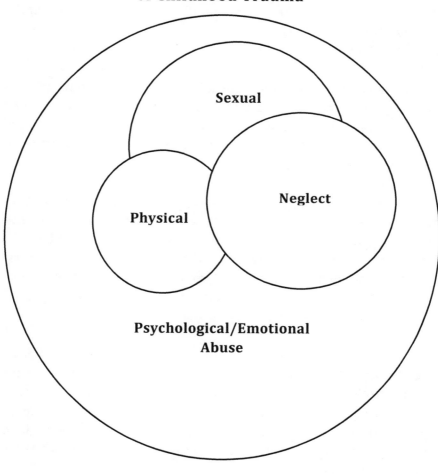

---

[7] Each may be overt, covert (subtle), or both. Estimated and expanded from Muenzenmaier et al. 1993, Anda et al. 2002 [173]

THE PROCESS OF WOUNDING

1) Previously traumatized and wounded themselves, the child's parents feel inadequate, bad and unfulfilled, i.e., they feel hurt, shame, confusion and emptiness.

2) They unconsciously project those charged feelings onto others, especially onto their spouse and their vulnerable children. They may also exhibit and project grandiosity (e.g., "I always know what's best for you!" —when they don't). They look outside of themselves to feel whole.

3) In a need to stabilize the parents and to survive, the child denies that the parents are inadequate and mistreating. With the unhealthy boundaries that the child has learned from its parents and others, the child internalizes (takes in, accepts) the parents' projected inadequacy and shame. A common fantasy is that, "If I'm really good and perfect, they will love me and they won't reject or abandon me." The child idealizes the parents.

4) The child's vulnerable true self [8] is wounded so often, that to protect that self it defensively submerges ("splits off") deep within the unconscious part of its psyche. The child goes into hiding (Figure 3.1 on page 28). The "child in hiding" represents what may appear at first to be a way that helps us to survive. Its downside is that going into hiding and staying there keeps us alienated from the power of knowing and being our true self. By its true self going into hiding, the child becomes alienated from its present

---

[8] Other terms for the real self include true self, our true identity, existential self, heart, soul, and child within. This is opposed to the false self, also called ego or co-dependent self, which is an assistant or kind of "side kick" to the true self that can help us negotiate our family and world. (I use the term ego here in a more simple and expanded way from its conventional understandings, wherein it was previously viewed erroneously, perhaps with some confusion, as being both true self and false self.)

experience in a number of ways—and from past experiences by forgetting much of the traumas that actually happened.

5) The child becomes alienated from its inner life—which includes emotionally painful responses to abuse and neglect, such as fear, shame, grief and anger. The child also becomes unaware of what is happening with others: "Daddy's not drunk. He was so tired he fell asleep on the lawn."

When our true self is in hiding—which it does to try to survive an otherwise unbearable life experience—it is unable to encode its impactful memories into its long-term memory in a conscious and currently useful way. Yet, paradoxically it somehow stores these memories in its unconscious mind as "old tapes," unfinished business, stored painful energy or ungrieved grief, much of which the object relations psychologists call "object representations" [9]

6) When children are not allowed to express their grief in a healthy way, their true self will try to find its own way out and express its painful experiences, like an enclosed abscess that is waiting to drain. But **unexpressed pain may** be stored as toxic energy and may **then manifest** in their life **as** a physical, **mental**, **emotional** or spiritual **disorder** or **illness**, or more usually as a

---

[9] The establishment of the false self (ego) may include some aspects of traumatic forgetting (dissociative amnesia) that are accompanied by the behaviors and responses that allow us to try to stabilize the family and avoid further abuse. As kinds of traumatic memory distortions, these characteristically involve a dissociation and/or censoring of some aspects of the traumas, such as the emotional pain of the abuse, and may involve the amnesia for some, most or even all of the traumatic experiences, and the substitution of an idealized past for the truth. [35,36,168] See Chapter 13 on page 170 for more details.

combination of these. Another term for this repeated attempt to express its trauma and grief is *repetition compulsion* [67,93,173].

7) The true self continues to take in whatever else it is told—both verbally and nonverbally—about itself and about others, and stores it in its **unconscious (mostly)** and its conscious mind (sometimes and to some degree).

Figure 3.1 The Child Goes into Hiding

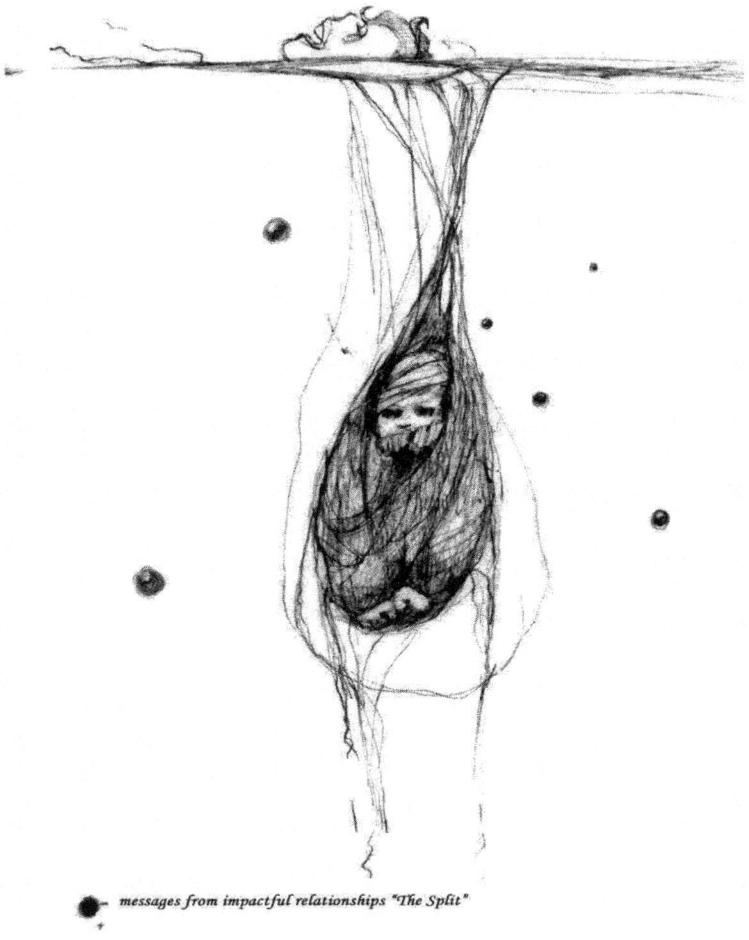

messages from impactful relationships "The Split"

8) What it takes in are messages from major and impactful relationships, primarily parents, but these may also include siblings, grandparents, clergy, and other authority and parent figures. The experiential representations of these relationships in the unconscious memory that continue to affect these children as adults are called "objects" or "object representations" by the object relations theorists and clinicians. These messages and representations are *laden with feelings*, and tend to occur in "part-objects" (e.g., good parent, bad parent, aggressive child, shy child, and so on). The more self-destructive messages tend to be deposited in the false self or "internal saboteur," also described as the internalized rejecting or otherwise mistreating parent. 67,93,173,181

9) Hurting, confused and feeling unable to run their own life, the child/person eventually turns that function over to the false self.

10) A tension builds. The true self is always striving to come alive and to evolve. At the same time, the "negative ego" (the destructive part of the false self) attacks the true self, thus forcing it to stay submerged (Figure 3.1 above), keeping self-esteem low. Also, the child's grieving of its losses and traumas is not supported. Because of all of the above, the child's development is disordered and boundaries become unhealthy. [10] This resulting "psychopathology" or "lesion" has been called a "schizoid compromise" and a "splitting off of the true self." 67,93,173,181 The outcome can be a developmental delay, arrest or failure.

---

[10] Children and adolescents need to be given and taught healthy boundaries, which help them feel safe and function better. Parents who are loose or inconsistent with their own and others' boundaries are subtly traumatizing their child. 96,167

11) Some **results** include **"mental illness,"** often with traumatic forgetting, chronic emptiness, fear, sadness and confusion, and periodic explosions of self-destructive and other destructive behavior—both impulsive and compulsive—that allow some temporary release of the tension and a glimpse of the true self.

12) The consequences of the continued emptiness and/or repeated destructive behavior keep the true self stifled or submerged. Not living from and as their real self—with a full awareness of their experiences—and with no safe people to talk to about them, often dissociated and numb, in order to survive they may forget, dissociate or otherwise shut out most of their painful experiences (dissociative or traumatic amnesia). [35,36,168]

13) The child/person maintains a low sense of self-esteem, remains unhappy, yet wishes and seeks fulfillment. Compulsions and addictions (and other repetition compulsions) can provide temporary release, but lead to more suffering and ultimately block recovery, fulfillment and serenity.

RECOVERY

14) Recovery and growth are discovering and gently unearthing the true self (real self, child within, true identity, core being) so that it can exist and express itself in a healthy way, day to day. It also means restructuring the false self or ego to become a more flexible assistant ("positive ego") to the true self. Some other results of working a full recovery program are growth, creativity and aliveness.

15) Such self-discovery and recovery is usually best accomplished gradually and in the presence of safe, compassionate, skilled and supportive people. Recovery is a cyclical process, and while it has its moments of peace, joy and liberating self-discovery, it is also

common to experience periods in which confusion, **symptoms that appear to be manifestations of "mental illness"** and suffering intensify. Participation in supportive recovery groups teaches the person how to deal with these cycles as they experience how others deal with their emotions, problems and with their growth and accomplishments in the recovery process. With commitment to and active participation in recovery, this healing process may take from three to five years or more [164,165,175].

16) By listening, sharing and reflecting in a safe environment, the trauma survivor begins slowly to remember what happened. They begin to reconstruct the physical, mental and emotional unhealed fragments of their memory that were previously buried deep within their unconscious mind. This crucial and healing kind of uncovering and remembering involves a process that evolves slowly over time.

17) During recovery the trauma survivor **learns** to **experience**, **express** and **tolerate emotional pain**, and by doing so experience its (their emotional pain's) movement and transient nature. This is the opposite of being overwhelmed by and mired in the stagnant pain and numbness of depression, which is commonly accompanied by bothersome anxiety (i.e., fear).

In the next chapter I will further describe the process of trauma by reviewing what we know about how it effects our self-esteem and our ability to have a healthy relationship or "attachment" growing up with our parents and eventually living and working with others. I will also continue to address more on the process of recovery and healing.

4   The Effects of Shame

BEING TOLD THAT WE ARE "MENTALLY ILL" AND MISTREATED
FOR OUR PAIN USUALLY DEEPENS OUR ALREADY DISABLING
SHAME

And there is a way out.

Having summarized these dynamics of trauma in Chapter 3, each trauma survivor also has their own experience and effects. Two of the more unifying and core experiences of trauma are the effect of PTSD, and a pervasive, underlying belief and feeling of shame. Shame has many guises, which I describe throughout this chapter. If shame is the umbrella, its spokes are low self-esteem or self-worth, shyness, easy embarrassment, self-deprecation, self-hate, at times the seeming opposites of arrogance and/or grandiosity and more, as I elaborate below. It reflects a decreased awareness of our true self, which we usually have lost. Our lost selfhood is probably the most hurtful effect of repeated childhood trauma. Burdened with shame, we may not be able to care for ourself in a healthy way.

CHARACTERISTICS

Shame is an uncomfortable or painful feeling that we experience when—consciously or unconsciously—we sense that a part of us is defective, bad, incomplete, rotten, phony, inadequate or a failure. In contrast to **guilt**, where we feel bad from *doing* something wrong, we feel **shame** from believing that we are *being* something wrong or bad. Thus guilt seems to be correctable or forgivable, whereas there may seem to be no way out of shame.

Our true self feels the shame and when appropriate can express it in a healthy way to safe and supportive people. Our false self, on

32

the other hand, pretends not to have the shame and would never tell anyone about it.

We *all* have some shame. Its only healthy form is humility.[176] Shame is universal to the human condition. If we do not work through it and then let go of it, shame tends to accumulate and often burdens us more over time, until we become its victim. In addition to feeling defective or inadequate, shame makes us believe that others can see through us, through our facade, and into our defectiveness. Shame feels hopeless: that no matter what we do, we cannot correct it. With shame we feel isolated and lonely, as though we are the only one who has it.

We may say, "I'm afraid to tell you about my shame because if I do, you'll think I'm bad, and I can't stand hearing how bad I am." And so not only do I keep it to myself, but I often block it out or pretend that it is not there.

I may even *disguise* my shame as if it were some other feeling or action and then *project* that *onto other people*, including those who are close to me. Some of these feelings and actions that may cover up, *mask* or *bind* our shame include:

- **Anger** • **Resentment** • **Contempt** • **Rage** • **Attack** • **Blame**
- **Control** • **Neglect/withdrawal** • **Abandonment**
- **Compulsive behavior** • **Perfectionism**

And when I feel or act out any of these guises of shame, it serves a useful purpose for my co-dependent or false self—acting as a defense against my feeling ashamed. But, even though I may defend myself well against my shame, it can still be seen by others, e.g., when I hang my head, slump down, avoid eye contact, wear sunglasses indoors, or make apologies for having my feelings, needs, wants, and rights. I may even feel somewhat nauseated, cold, withdrawn and alienated. But no matter how well I may

33

defend myself and others against it, my shame will not go away—unless I **learn what** it is, **name it accurately** when I encounter it, **experience** it more **consciously** and **share** it with **safe** and **supportive others**. [164,165] The best place to do this is in ongoing individual or group therapy and self-help fellowship meetings.

CASE HISTORY 4.1 example of the guise that our shame can take happened in group therapy when Jim, a 35-year-old accountant began to tell the group about his relationship with his father who lives in another state "Every time we talk on the phone he tries to judge me. I get so confused that I want to hang up." Jim talked more and interacted with the group who asked him what feelings were coming up right now. He had some difficulty being aware of and identifying his feelings, and made little eye contact with the group. "I'm just confused. I always wanted to be perfect around him. And I never could do it to his satisfaction." He talked further, and the group asked him again what feelings were coming up for him right now. "I feel some fear, some hurt and I guess I'm a little angry." As a group leader, I also asked him if he might be feeling some shame as though he were somehow an inadequate person. He said, "No. Why would you think of that?" I pointed out that his drive to be perfect, his avoidance of eye contact, and the way he described his relationship with his father suggested to me that he was feeling some shame. A tear came to his eye, and he said he would have to think about it. His father continued to emotionally abuse him.

WHERE DOES OUR SHAME COME FROM?

Our shame seems to come from what we do with the negative messages, negative affirmations, beliefs and rules that we hear, see and experience as we grow up in a troubled family and world. We hear and experience these abuses from our parents, parent figures, and other people in authority, such as teachers, bosses and clergy. These messages basically tell us that we are somehow not all right, not okay. That our feelings, our needs, our true self or child within is not acceptable.

Over and over, we hear messages like "shame on you!" "You're so bad!" "You're not good enough!" We hear them so often, and from people on whom we are so dependant and to whom we are so vulnerable, that we believe them. And so we incorporate or internalize them into our very being.

As if that were not enough, the wound is compounded by negative rules that stifle and prohibit the otherwise healthy healing and needed expression of our pains. Rules like "Don't feel," "Don't cry" and "Children are to be seen and not heard." And so not only do we learn that we are bad, but that we are not to talk openly about any of it.

However, these negative rules are often inconsistently enforced. The result? Difficulty in trusting rule-makers and authority figures, and we feel fear, guilt, and more shame. And where do our parents learn these negative messages and rules? Most likely from their parents and other authority figures. This is another example of childhood trauma (here as emotional abuse) being transmitted from one generation to the next. (See page 47 of my book *Healing the Child Within* for a list of negative rules and messages commonly heard in troubled families.)

THE SHAME-BASED FAMILY

When everyone in a dysfunctional family comes from and communicates with others from a base or common practice of shame or shaming, it can be described as shame-based.

Parents in such a family did not have their needs met as infants and children and usually as they continue into adulthood as well. They often use their children to meet many of these unmet needs [104,164,165].

Shame-based families often, though not always, have a **secret**. This secret may span all kinds of "shameful" events or conditions, from family violence to sexual abuse to alcoholism to having been in a concentration camp or having a relative who was. Or the secret may be as subtle as a lost job, a lost promotion or a lost relationship. Keeping such secrets *disables* all members of the family, *whether or not they know* the secret. This is because being secretive prevents the *expression* of questions, concern and feelings (such as fear, anger, shame and guilt). And the family thus cannot communicate freely. And the true self/child within each family member remains stifled— unable to grow and develop.

DATA ON SHAME

Data is/are a collection of numbers, characters, images or other variables about things that we can compile and use to help us answer questions. While few researchers have looked for it, nearly all of those who did look found shame to be significantly present in the trauma survivors that they evaluated. In 31 data based reports that I found, the authors called it low self-esteem, which is also a DSM-IV diagnostic criterion for "depression"—which itself is overwhelmingly associated with and likely caused by repeated childhood trauma. But more important, *shame itself* is a frequent, if not universal, effect of repeated childhood and later trauma.

Using multiple and varied research methods, these 31 studies by independent authors studying diverse populations reported that among 6,329 people, low self-esteem was a common and important finding among the trauma survivors. It is thus useful to include an evaluation of a person's self-esteem and if appropriate, address it in their recovery plan. Shame (low self-esteem) is a common and debilitating long-term effect of repeated childhood trauma. It blocks our motivation to heal ("I'm not worthy," "I don't deserve to get better, "I'm bad"). I summarize some effective ways to address it at the end of this chapter and in other books [165,173,174].

ATTACHMENT FINDINGS – THE EARLIEST TRAUMAS

The effects of childhood trauma hurt, and they are many and varied. Since the 1930s, clinicians and researchers have made countless observations that have substantiated the above patterns and dynamics on the process of wounding. Over the past 30 years numerous researchers have looked at the behavior of 11- to 16-month-old infants when they are exposed to a specific stressor. Most people cannot remember what happened for them at this time. Bear with me while I summarize.

Called the "strange situation," they looked at the way children react when their mother leaves them with a stranger briefly and then returns. Based on their results in 13 reports published from 1981 through 1993, they have found four common infant reactions. The first child reaction is **ideal**. It results from having a mother who is sensitive and appropriately attentive and responsive in her long-term care of her child. When stressed in this experimental way, the infant rapidly seeks the attachment figure (the mother), and when she returns, tends to be easily soothed, comforted and reassured by her, and is thereby soon ready to explore the environment again. [173] Called a ***secure attachment***, this kind differs from the other three types of infant attachment reactions when they have been previously traumatized or neglected outside of the experimental situation. These reactions may be a part of the early experience of many survivors of childhood trauma. All three have a fearful or anxious attachment with their mother, which I summarize in Table 7.4 on page 85 of *The Truth about Depression*. If the **mother** has usually been either rejecting or intrusive ("smothering"), neglecting, erratic or abusive, the **child** usually responds to the "strange situation" with avoidance, aggression, clinging, or freezes in confusion.

These "attachment" reactions represent snapshots of the early healthy and unhealthy parent-child relationship and have provided us with more understanding of how early trauma may affect a child. When they are known, child protection service workers and clinicians can use these kinds of observations in their work. While some have criticized the limitations of attachment theory, I believe that these observations support some of the above-described dynamics, in part, of how the child gets wounded. This trauma dynamic sets the stage for a life of shame.

RISKY FAMILIES

Numerous studies report the prior trauma and its effects on the parents, parent figures, siblings and the child's other relatives. One example study: Goodwin and colleagues looked at 100 **mothers of** sexually and/or physically **abused children**, and found these mothers were 8 times more likely to have been sexually **abused themselves** as children, when compared to five hundred controls [64]. Based on their own prior wounding, these mothers may not have been able to protect their children from abuse, and thereby became co-abusers or enablers of the abuse (which I describe further in my book *Memory and Abuse*).

What other risk factors may predispose a family to abuse its children? Another example: Brown and colleagues looked carefully at this question and found 17 significant unhealthy characteristics of mothers that put their children at a high risk for being abused. They also found 3 unhealthy characteristics of fathers, 6 of the children and 5 of the family as a whole that predisposed to the presence of child abuse and neglect. These unhealthy characteristics were associated with risk factors of from 5 to 11.8 times those found among the control or "normal" samples (page 87 of *The Truth about Depression*). These are significantly high numbers. Impaired, troubled or disordered parents put their children at especially high risk for being abused or neglected by themselves and others. To help break the trans-generational cycle of abuse, we need to take these data seriously and develop effective ways to use this information to prevent future childhood trauma.

RECOVERY AIDS FOR HEALING SHAME: PART 1

In my work assisting trauma survivors in their recovery I have observed an almost universal finding of low self-esteem among them. The belief and painful feeling of shame declares that "I am bad, not enough, flawed, inadequate, imperfect and even rotten at my core." Shame appears to be taught and learned, repeatedly implanted by abusers, which their victims incorporate into their beings. This subtle yet toxic process often begins at birth and can continue as repeated child abuse, and more traumas may be repeated throughout an adult's life. Active shame blocks healing.

Shame v Guilt - *in Review* A recovery program can slowly address and heal the effects of trauma, including the shame. Primary in healing shame is first to **name it** accurately, in whatever guise it may appear (Figure 4.1 summarizes many of them). **Naming things accurately** gives us **personal power**. In review from above: it is important to differentiate shame from guilt. Sometimes confused with shame, **guilt** is a painful feeling that comes from making a mistake, *doing* something wrong—or not doing it right. We can heal guilt by apologizing or making amends to the person we may have wronged, and, if appropriate, perhaps even asking for forgiveness. Guilt is about doing or not doing.

Figure 4.1 Guises of Shame

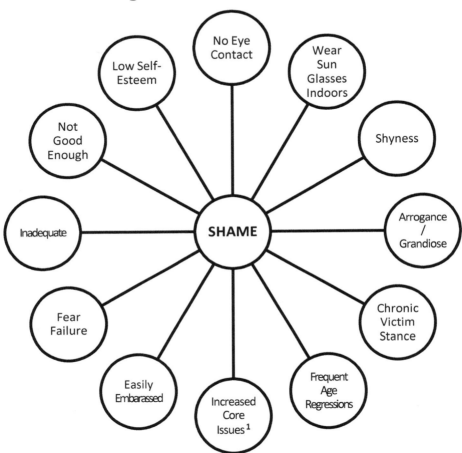

[1] e.g., high tolerance for inappropriate behavior, difficulty handling conflict, fear of abandonment, and difficulty giving and receiving love.

Shame is about being or not being. In guilt, we have *done* something wrong which we can more easily correct. In shame, we feel and even think as though we *are* something wrong, and we can see no way to correct it. Often fostered by some organized religions as "original sin," we feel as though we are born defective and bad. From this collective shaming trauma, our false self/ego then maintains the shame. As one patient said, "I have a tape recorder in my head that reminds me of how bad I am."

Another said, "There is this constant broadcast in the pit of my being telling me I'm not good enough." Shame can be so pervasive that it can stop people from going into recovery because they believe they don't deserve to, or that they will never feel better.

Case History 4.2: Sharon was a forty-four-year-old woman who came to me complaining of a strong and painful sense of insecurity. She had been physically abused and neglected throughout her childhood. In group therapy over time, as she worked on her relationship and trauma issues, she realized that it was really shame or low self-esteem that was robbing her of "being able to feel secure." She often described her "battle" as trying to box her way out of a canvas bag. No matter how hard she struggled, she couldn't see and free herself. Over time, she shared her burdensome feeling and experience of shame with the therapy group and revealed it from many different angles. Eventually she was able to grieve for her painful and lost childhood. With compassion and acceptance from the group, Sharon eventually was able to feel compassion for herself, realizing how severely she had been treated. She told the group that the voices inside her head telling her how bad she was weren't quite so loud anymore, and she could now often hear her real self as soothing her.

A major way to heal shame is to **share our experience** of it with **safe people**. [164,165] An effective way to do that is to tell our story or narrative, bit by bit, of what happened to us in our trauma experiences. This process may be accomplished in individual therapy or counseling, during heart-to-heart talks with a trusted and safe friend, and in group therapy or a self-help group. Each time that we share our shame with safe people, we express it, and thereby expel it outside of ourself. By doing so, we paradoxically own that we experienced it, and then we can get rid of it. **We release what we know, understand and express**. Shame usually takes such repeated sharing over a long time to heal.

While there are some data-based studies that show an overall improvement using individual and group therapy, most of the experience on healing shame is anecdotal, although it is based on decades of careful observation on countless trauma survivors as they heal. [174] These reports also validate ways to help heal shame from a rich and consistent perspective.

If someone **believes** that they are **mentally ill**, doing so may **aggravate** and compound that shame. Shame will likely rear its subtle but ugly head numerous times during recovery. However, participating in a recovery program will eventually affirm our inherent goodness as we heal from the toxic effects of shame.

To start this chapter I said that two of the more unifying and core experiences of trauma are the effect of PTSD, and a pervasive, underlying belief and feeling of shame. I also said that our lost selfhood is probably the most hurtful effect of repeated childhood trauma. Because PTSD, shame and lost selfhood accompany one another so pervasively and mask as "mental illness" so often, I will now describe the basic features of PTSD in the next chapter.

5 Post-Traumatic Stress Disorder

"When I felt burdened by fear or depression, I had to remind myself that I wasn't crazy. I just had PTSD."
—John, 41 years-old, 2 years in recovery

I have found post-traumatic stress disorder (PTSD) to be the most accurate, inclusive and potentially useful of all of the *DSM* (the American Psychiatric Association's "bible" of mental illness/disorders) diagnostic categories. Its **accuracy** begins with the fact that many of the common mental disorders are strongly associated with, and often caused by, repeated childhood and other trauma. At the least they are often aggravated by it, as shown throughout this and two of my prior books. [173,174]

It's **inclusiveness** rests in the fact that PTSD's diverse symptoms can be manifested and thus masqueraded by several other common disorders, including *depression, substance abuse/chemical dependence, anxiety* and *panic disorder, somatization disorder,* and *dissociative* and at times *psychotic disorders* and more (see Table 6.1 on page 57). That is, any of these may be an erroneous diagnosis, because the person actually has PTSD instead.

PTSD also commonly is a co-occuring condition (also called "co-morbid" in clinical language) with any one or more of these. And its **usefulness** lies in its ability to reframe and at times clarify a common cause of human suffering as being caused simply by unmetabolized (unprocessed, unreleased and unhealed) trauma effects (which are all the bothersome symptoms and emotional pain that may have led you to think you might be "mentally ill"). Knowing about it thereby frees sufferers from the fear, guilt, and shame that they are somehow responsible— and bad, sick, crazy or stupid—by showing that they are instead, just wounded.

Trauma occurs when any act, event or experience harms or decreases the physical, sexual, mental, emotional or spiritual integrity and functionality of our true self. Simple upsetting or disrupting of it is not usually enough to cause actual harm, unless it is *repeated* over time and is of *human origin*. And if we are vulnerable, i.e., if our true self is already wounded or hurt from prior trauma, then we may be more likely to develop additional or more severe symptoms and signs of post-traumatic stress when we are exposed to additional trauma.

The American Psychiatric Association has described a spectrum of psychosocial *stressors* which range from mild to severe (Table 5.1). These are but a *few examples* of traumas, but are useful ones to consider, since several psychiatrist and psychologist authors ranked them according to their estimated levels of severity.

The three main B/C/D groups of symptoms in PTSD include *re-experiencing* of the trauma in various ways, a persistent *avoidance* of stimuli that are associated with the trauma, and persistent symptoms of increased *arousal* (Table 5.2). In addition to the trauma history, there is also usually a **numbing** of the person's awareness of their inner life, especially their feelings, and frequently some degree of **traumatic forgetting** (Figure 5.1).
Difficulty remembering aspects of traumatic experiences is so common in PTSD that it is used in at least ten of its approximately twenty diagnostic criteria in the DSM-IV. Indeed, rather than being the exception after experiencing trauma, as some skeptics claim, memory difficulties tend more often to be the rule, which many clinicians and researchers have described [35,36,168].

Remembering what happened in our traumatic experience: This remembering is not simply cognitive, but is also experiential. As we heal, we re-experience the trauma with increasing awareness in a constructive, non-dissociated consciousness,

44

Table 5.1 Severity Rating of Psychosocial Stressors
(from DSM-3)

Severity: *Child/Adolescent* Examples	*Adult* Examples
1. **None** No apparent psychological stressor	No apparent psychological stressor
2. **Minimal** Vacation with family	Minor violation of the law; small bank loan
3. **Mild** Change in schoolteacher; new school year	Argument with neighbor; change in work hours
4. **Moderate** Chronic parental fighting; change to new school; illness of close relative; sibling birth	New career; death of close friend; pregnancy
5. **Severe** Death of peer; divorce of parents; arrest; hospitalization; persistent separation; and harsh parental discipline	Serious illness in self or family; major financial loss; marital separation; birth of child and harsh parental discipline
6. **Extreme** Death of parent or sibling; repeated physical or sexual abuse	Death of close relative; divorce
7. **Catastrophic** Multiple family deaths	Devastating natural disaster; concentration camp experience

which evolves during the recovery process (more discussion in Chapter 13). See page 212 in Appendix II for further information on PTSD, especially on Category A in Table 5.2 on the next page.

GUISES OF PTSD

PTSD is a *great masquerader*, similar to alcoholism and other **chemical dependence** (next chapter). It can **mimic** and present as **any** one or more of the **most common mental illnesses described in the *DSM*, elsewhere and in this book.**

Table 5.2. PTSD Diagnostic Criteria from DSM-4 (309.81)

A. The person has been exposed to a traumatic event [or events] in which both of the following have been present:	1. the person has experienced, witnessed, or been confronted with an event or events that involve actual or threatened death or serious injury, or a threat to the physical integrity of oneself or others. 2. the person's response involved intense fear, helplessness, or horror. {My experience is that these 2 criteria are the least important of A - F]
B. The **traumatic event** is persistently **re-experienced** in at least one of the following ways:	1. recurrent and intrusive distressing recollections of the event, including images, thoughts, or perceptions. 2. recurrent distressing dreams of the event. 3. acting or feeling as if the traumatic event were recurring (includes a sense of reliving the experience, illusions, hallucinations, and dissociative flashback episodes, including those that occur upon awakening or when intoxicated) 4. intense psychological distress at exposure to internal or external cues that symbolize or resemble an aspect of the traumatic event 5. physiologic reactivity upon exposure to internal or external cues that symbolize or resemble an aspect of the traumatic event
C. Persistent **avoidance** of stimuli associated with the trauma and **numbing** of general responsiveness (not present before the trauma), as indicated by at least three of the following:	1. efforts to avoid thoughts, feelings, or conversations associated with the trauma 2. efforts to avoid activities, places, or people that arouse recollections of the trauma 3. inability to recall an important aspect of the trauma 4. markedly diminished interest or participation in significant activities 5. feeling of detachment or estrangement from others 6. restricted range of affect (e.g., have loving feelings) 7. sense of a foreshortened future (e.g., does not expect to have a career, marriage, children, or a normal life span)
D. Persistent symptoms of increased **arousal** (not present before the trauma), as indicated by at least two of the following:	1. difficulty falling or staying asleep 2. irritability or outbursts of anger 3. difficulty concentrating, 4. hypervigilance 5. exaggerated startle response. [**Final 2 Criteria:**] **E.** Duration of the disturbance (symptoms in B, C, and D) is more than one month **F.** The disturbance causes **clinically significant distress** or **impairment** in social, occupational, or other important areas of functioning.

Figure 5.1 Major Components of PTSD

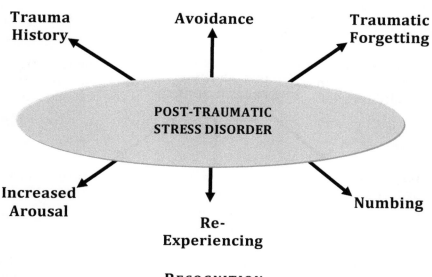

RECOGNITION

PTSD may occur in **multiple** and varied **guises** and **associations,** from **anxiety** to **depression** to **dissociative** and **personality disorders** to **psychosis.** Thus, health professionals and others should maintain a high index of suspicion for the possible presence of PTSD among most of the people they evaluate and assist. *Have yours done so with you*? If you are a clinician, do you look for it?

PTSD has presented itself in many guises throughout history. In the late 1800s and early 1900s, during the time of Janet, Freud and their colleagues, it was called *hysteria* and was seen more often in traumatized young women. During World Wars I and 2 it was seen most often in young men, and was called *shell shock* or *combat neurosis.* And when people are taken hostage or kept and abused in concentration camps, what usually results is also PTSD (Figure 5.2 on the next page).

Figure 5.2. **Guises of PTSD over Recent History**

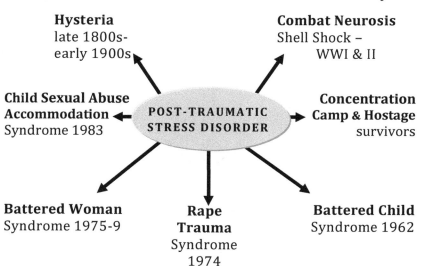

Even though children have been physically and otherwise abused for millennia, we did not begin to recognize *battered child* syndrome until about 1962, when it was first described, another guise of the disorder. Twelve to fifteen years later, two more variations of PTSD were described: the *rape trauma* syndrome in 1974 and the *battered woman* syndrome in 1975 to 1979. One of the more recently recognized guises is the *child sexual abuse accommodation* syndrome, described by psychiatrist Roland Summit in 1983. [152] PTSD is also commonly seen among young and adult *children of dysfunctional families* and occurs often in people of all ages with other *mental* and *physical* disorders.

While these guises may have various things in common, including their association with PTSD, people who are afflicted with any of them tend to be laden with fear, shame and guilt. *Fear* because of the terror of the unhealed original trauma. *Shame* because of the factors discussed in the last chapter and that our political, social and helping professional systems are generally so unaware of what to do to help survivors of childhood trauma. Many of these authorities may be fearful of facing their own wounds that they tend to project their own unhealed shame onto the victims of these many kinds of abuse. Rather than assist and help, not doing so often hinders and re-traumatizes. And **guilt** because we as survivors feel that we somehow *caused* the abuse, even though we did not.

Central to all of the above is that when we are traumatized and then naturally and appropriately try to express our resulting pain, in these dysfunctional systems—home, school, most doctors, clinic, hospital, politicians, street, with peers—we are repeatedly *invalidated* for doing so. Being invalidated not only blocks and often destroys our natural mechanisms for healing, but it frequently inflicts a double trauma on the victim. Most all of the *invalidations* (whether individual or collective) *against our genuine attempts to heal* are thus just **another** kind of **trauma**—known as **re-traumatization,** also called **revictimization** (discussed in some detail on page 207 of *The Truth about Mental Illness*).

The *intensity* of the trauma, *characteristics* or *kind* of trauma, and our *subjective response* to it, including our *opportunity* and *ability* to *process* and *heal from* the traumatic experience, are all important in influencing the personal and clinical effects that result from the trauma. To have been mistreated by our parents or another person who is supposed to be protective of our welfare and well-being is traumatic enough. But to heap on top of that trauma their blocking of our ability to express and grieve the traumatic experience and heal ourselves is equally as traumatic. Other than their original traumas, survivors tend also to experience more stressful life events and re-victimization than others, which I describe in *The Truth about Mental Illness*. Some of these latter people may have *complex* PTSD.

SIDEBAR —A NOTE ABOUT STRESS

Stress is neither "good" nor "bad." However, depending on how we choose to use it, stress may be positive or negative in our life. It can thus be growth-inducing, or it can cause illness and suffering, or both. Transient stress is usually short-lived, especially if it is dissipated with muscle action or with another fairly quick and ameliorating response, and thus itself is not damaging. Such a response has been called eustress (Seyle 1974, Pelletier 1977, Cox 1979, Nuernberger 1981, Girdano & Everly 1979). However chronic stress, also called distress (Seyle 1974), occurs when the person has an incomplete and thus unhealthy response to a demand, and tension remains and accumulates.

Distress is a prolongation and a continuation of acute stress and may accumulate and linger indefinitely. When stress is prolonged in this manner, it can fatigue the body, often targeting certain organs. These target organs vary among individuals. Chronic stress and distress can continue for months or years without the person knowing or feeling it.

Physiologically, the stress response consists of a nonspecific arousal caused by stimulation of the adrenergic or sympathetic nervous system. Here the hypothalamus releases corticotropin releasing hormone (CRH), which stimulates the pituitary gland to release ACTH, which then causes the adrenal gland to release cortisol, aldosterone, and norepinephrine and epinephrine (adrenalin) into the bloodstream. The blood glucose rises, as do serum triglycerides and free fatty acids. Often erroneously called "stress," the stimulus that causes the arousal is more accurately called a "stressor." Psychiatric drugs cause an internal stress and distress which I describe in Chapter 7.

COMPLEX PTSD

Complex PTSD (also called Complex Stress Disorder or Disorder of Extreme Stress Not Otherwise Specified [DESNOS]) is another, yet *extreme*, guise or variant of PTSD that is commonly seen among trauma survivors who were exposed to repeated trauma, especially during childhood. In addition to the above usual symptoms of PTSD, these people may also experience increased episodes of *dissociation*, marked *relationship difficulties*, *re-victimization*, *somatization*, extreme *disrupted feelings* and *emotions*, and a *lost sense of self* and *meaning* in their life.

As clinical and research trauma psychiatrist Judith Herman described it concisely, the person with complex PTSD usually has a history of subjection to totalitarian control over a prolonged period (months to years). Examples outside the family include hostages, prisoners of war, concentration-camp survivors and survivors of some religious cults. Examples also include those subjected to totalitarian systems in family life, such as survivors of domestic battering, childhood physical or sexual abuse, and organized sexual exploitation. The specific findings may be: 1) Alterations in affect (feelings and emotions) regulation, including: persistent dysphoria (emotional pain), chronic suicidal preoccupation, self-injury, explosive or extremely inhibited anger (these may alternate), compulsive or extremely inhibited sexuality (may alternate); 2) Alterations in consciousness, including: amnesia or hyperamnesia for traumatic events, transient dissociative episodes, depersonalization/derealization, reliving traumatic experiences, either in the form of intrusive post-traumatic stress disorder symptoms or as ruminative preoccupation; 3) Alterations in self-perception, including: sense of helplessness or paralysis of initiative, shame, guilt, and self-blame, sense of defilement or stigma, sense of complete difference from others (may include sense of specialness, utter aloneness, belief no other person can understand, or nonhuman identity); 4) Alterations in perception of perpetrator, including: preoccupation with relationship with perpetrator (includes preoccupation with revenge), unrealistic attribution of total power to perpetrator (caution: victim's assessment of power realities may be more realistic than clinician's), idealization or paradoxical gratitude, sense of special or supernatural relationship, acceptance of belief system or rationalizations of perpetrator; 5) Alterations in relations with others, including: isolation and withdrawal, disruption in intimate relationships, repeated search for rescuer (may alternate with isolation and withdrawal), persistent distrust, repeated failures of self-protection; 6) Alterations in systems of meaning: loss of sustaining faith, sense of hopelessness and despair. (Complex Post-Traumatic Stress Disorder Recommended DSM diagnostic criteria, from *Trauma and Recovery* by Judith Herman, 1992 Basic Books)

Many brain and hormonal abnormalities occur from early repeated trauma, and appear to cause difficulties with memory, learning, and regulating impulses and emotions. All of these trauma effects may contribute to severe behavioral difficulties (such as impulsivity, aggression, sexual acting out, eating disorders, alcohol/drug abuse and self-destructive actions), emotional regulation difficulties (such as intense rage, depression or panic) and mental difficulties (such as extremely scattered thoughts, dissociation and amnesia). As adults, people with complex PTSD are often diagnosed with depression, personality or dissociative disorders, or psychosis. Their recovery and improvement often takes much longer, may progress at a much slower rate, often interspersed with frequent crises, and requires a sensitive and structured treatment program delivered by a trauma specialist. [43,71]

HISTORY 2.1

Marta was a forty-three-year-old woman who came to me for assistance with a painful life in chaos. She had recurring depression, anxiety and repeated failed relationships and job difficulties. She had severe premenstrual syndrome, recurrent asthma, smoked two packs of cigarettes a day and had been raped twice in the past ten years. She had been diagnosed with depression, borderline personality disorder, "bipolar disorder" and had been hospitalized several times for these. She had been treated with numerous antidepressant drugs and benzodiazepine sedatives with little or no improvement. Five years ago, during her last relationship with a man, she felt safe enough to remember increasingly more details of being brutally physically and psychologically abused by her father and neglected by her mother as a child. She had partial memories of having been sexually abused by her father and another unidentified man. None of her recent clinicians had addressed her trauma history, nor had any of them before that inquired about possible trauma.

I saw her weekly in individual psychotherapy for six months, during which time she had such marked swings in her emotions and ability to function that she was unable to join our trauma-focused therapy group. She had to be hospitalized twice for brief psychotic episodes, at which time the attending psychiatrist made a provisional diagnosis of "bipolar disorder," although over the next few years she did not have another psychotic or manic episode. Because of her continuing severe premenstrual syndrome pain, her gynecologist performed a hysterectomy and removed her ovaries, after which her mood swings improved enough for her to join our therapy group. Over the next three years, her chaotic and painful life began to improve, and at this point she has been able to keep a job and an ongoing relationship with a man for over a year, which, she says, is a record for her. She realizes that she has more issues to address.

Although the details may vary, Marta's story is typical for many people with complex PTSD. Before she could begin the long and difficult trauma effects healing work in a Stage Two recovery program, she first needed to stabilize in a Stage One program, during which she did a number of things to help herself stabilize (these stages are further described in Chapter 14 and summarized in Table 14.1 on pages 173 and following). These included stopping smoking cigarettes (one of the most difficult but helpful choices), improving her diet and nutrition, beginning an exercise program, seeing me in weekly individual psychotherapy sessions, and having appropriate attention given to her gynecological problem. It is unfortunate that most people with this very disruptive disorder of complex PTSD do not get the opportunity to heal their pain in a trauma-focused recovery program. Instead, many suffer through their personal and work lives, use the health care system much more than average, including frequent hospitalizations, while the health care and health insurance systems tend to ignore the role of trauma as a major causal factor in their mental and some physical illnesses.

VARIANTS OF PTSD

In my experience I have come to see 4 kinds or variants of PTSD, which I summarize in Table 5.3. Among the countless PTSD patients I have seen over the years, classical PTSD has been the most common, followed by the less common sub-variant kind and complex PTSD. I discuss the increasingly common Drug Stress Trauma Syndrome variant of PTSD in Chapter 7.

Table 5.3 Variants of PTSD

PTSD Variant	*Characteristics and Description*
PTSD Sub-variant [179]	Little, unclear or no memory of Category A trauma experiences or history. May fulfill less *DSM* diagnostic criteria than required for classical PTSD, yet patient usually has one or more trauma spectrum disorders and other trauma effects.
Classical PTSD [157]	Memory/awareness for enough trauma effects to fulfill *DSM* criteria for PTSD categories A – F
Complex PTSD [43,71]	Extreme variant after repeated severe trauma, especially during childhood. Commonly experience increased *dissociation,* marked *relationship difficulties, re-victimization, somatization,* extreme *disrupted feelings* and *emotions,* and a *lost sense of self* and *meaning.*
Drug Stress Trauma Syndrome (DSTS) [179]	An unknown minority % may have DSTS without having another PTSD variant. Needs data gathering. Many usually have another variant of PTSD *plus* DSTS [179]

PTSD and its variants, dimensions, and manifestations are so common and pervasive and they represent more than the simple description that the *DSM* psychiatric diagnosis codebook presents. Because of this fact, I will continue to describe PTSD further in its association with addictions in the next chapter and in several other parts of this book (pages 56 and following, including page 212 in Appendix II).

6   Alcoholism & Other Addictions: Their Role in Mental Illness

Addictions are a sleeping giant that routinely cause psychological and behavioral problems and symptoms that appear on the surface as "mental illness." Alcoholism, other drug dependence, and other addictions (which in this chapter I will refer to as simply *addictions*) play several roles in their interaction with what we call mental illness. Some of these roles include:

1) Like PTSD, addictions can mimic and masquerade as all of the common mental disorders and most of the less common ones. All people with emotional or behavior problems should be carefully screened for alcoholism, other drug dependence and other addictions.

2) Clinicians of all sorts, from physicians to nurses to psychologists and counselors frequently misdiagnose addictions as though they were mental illness and thereby mistreat these common conditions.

3) Most people with addictions have a history of repeated childhood and later trauma as shown in Table 1.2 on page 10, 6.2 on page 60 and in my books (2003 & 4), and subsequently

4) Many to most also have an underlying PTSD.

5) Once the addiction is stabilized for a time in a Stage One full recovery program, recovery work that *addresses the trauma effects* (Stage Two) can help prevent relapse of the addiction and maintain, expand and strengthen the person's ongoing recovery and quality of life.

6) Finally, there is no convincing data-based evidence that psychiatric drugs *cure* any addiction or any mental illness.

In this chapter I will summarize these and other ways that addictions—and PTSD—interact with mental illness.

ADDICTIONS MIMIC MENTAL ILLNESS

Active addictions can generate any or all of the spectrum of symptoms of mental illness, from anxiety to "depression" to dysfunctional behaviors to psychosis (Table 6.1). When an accurate diagnosis of an addiction is made and a Stage One abstinence-oriented full recovery program is begun, over the next weeks and months many of these psychological symptoms will usually decrease or stop. Those symptoms that remain may be due to a complex web of interactions among other factors or conditions that themselves can also mimic or masquerade as mental illness, as shown in Figure 6.1. Hallucinations, delusions, other psychotic

Table 6.1 Addictions (±PTSD) can present as any of –

Depression	Unstable emotions	Difficulty focusing "ADHD"	Hyper-active/ -vigilant
Low energy	Anger outbursts	Social detachment or estrangement	Flashbacks
Anxiety	Fears and phobias	Panic attacks	OCD-like symptoms
Insomnia	Nightmares	Dissociation	"Bipolar"

Trauma effects can also present as any of these and more, as described throughout this book and in *The Truth about Depression* and *The Truth about Mental Illness.*

symptoms, or more severe dysfunction are often due to Complex PTSD (a more severe form described in the previous chapter).

Figure 6.1 The Complex Web of Interactions among the Great Masqueraders of Mental Illness

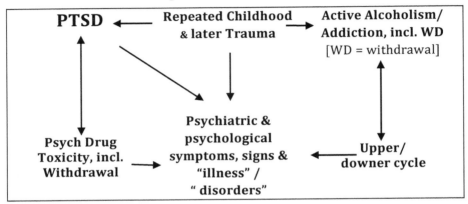

A problem is that too many people who know the symptomatic or troubled person, from clinicians to family, friends, teachers or co-workers, are *not usually aware* of these facts and associations. They commonly misdiagnose the distressed person as having one or more mental disorders and are quick to misprescribe or mis-recommend one or more psych *drugs*, which themselves *cause psychiatric symptoms* directly or indirectly through withdrawal and other toxic effects.

Having bought the claim that they have a "mental disorder," once the person begins taking a psych drug, they become entranced, confused, numbed and/or spellbound by the drug effects. Over time, they *become chemical dependent* on the psych drug—not usually because it makes them "high" in the ordinary sense—but because *when they try to stop* it, a disturbing *withdrawal reaction* occurs that is relieved only by returning to taking the drug, which then continues the drug's toxic effects and the vicious cycle of the need to stop the withdrawal.

A TRAUMA HISTORY

Most addicted people have a history of repeated childhood and later trauma. The scientific evidence for this fact is strong to overwhelming, as shown in Table 6.2. The bottom row of this table summarizes 272 studies (by independent researchers worldwide) on over a *half million* people that showed a *highly statistically significant* relationship between addictions and having a history of repeated childhood and later trauma. These researchers studied four different groups of people: 1) those people who lived in the *community* and 2) sought care in *clinical* settings; 3) other researchers also studied them over time (called *prospective* studies); finally they studied people who were 4) first identified as having an addiction (also called *index cases*). [173,174]

All four categories showed a strong to overwhelming link between having an addiction and a history of childhood and later trauma. In my long clinical experience, I have never seen a person with alcoholism or another drug addiction who grew up in a healthy family. An exception might be in the case of a person dependent on opiate drugs who has been treated for an injury-related pain problem, but who grew up in a healthy family.

Most authors and speakers who address the causal factors of these addictions do not include childhood trauma as a likelihood or even a possibility. Instead, they nearly always mention "genetically inherited" and a "brain chemistry" problem, when in truth the evidence is not convincing for these. [82,132,173,174] Thus, most of these authors' readers and listeners conclude in error that trauma is not a significant causal factor among these addictions, when in fact it is.

There *is* a need for taking a routine history for childhood and later trauma among all people with addictions and eventually to screen for PTSD in all of them. Doing so will likely help strengthen their recovery long term, since unaddressed trauma effects and related core recovery issues are common causes of relapse of addictions.

Table 6.2 Addictions and childhood trauma (CT)
Data-based published studies through 2003

Number Studies Years	Number of people studied	Addiction among CT survivors	Other effects Comments
1) **Alcoholism** 153 Studies 1942–2002	261,595 CT survivors v. controls	2–38x Clinical/Com; 1.2–10x Prospective; 30–84% CT in Index Cases	Multiple Co-morbidity common All support trauma link
2) **Eating disorders** (food addiction) 108 Studies 1986–2003	226,344 CT survivors v. controls	1.6–11x Clinical/Com; ↑ to 82% in Prospective; ↑ to 100% CT in Index Cases	↑ Co-morbidity All document CT link
3) **Nicotine addiction** 11 Studies 1992–2003	18,498 CT survivors v. controls	↑to 6x	↑Multiple co-morbidity
Summary[11] 272 studies 1942 - 2003	**506,437 CT survivors v. controls**	**1.6-38x Clinical/Com; 1.2–11x Prospective; 30–100% in Index Cases**	**Multiple Co-morbidity Common All support trauma link**

[11] Studies by Independent International Authors. Data from Whitfield CL: *The Truth about Mental Illness* 2004.

Charles L. Whitfield, M.D.

Another 16 studies (summarized in the second row in Table 6.3) evaluated a total of over 4,802 **addicted (chemical dependent) patients** and their controls from the general population. From 9 to 59% of those who were addicted had PTSD (compared with the far less 1.5 to 12% of PTSD found in the general population). Most authors noted that even with these highly statistically significant differences, these results probably *underestimate* the percentage of chemical dependent patients who also had PTSD, which I have found during my decades-long career assisting these patients.

Their active addiction's **high-risk life style** also exposes them to **continued traumas** that both worsen the PTSD and often trigger its relapse. And in a vicious cycle, relapses of PTSD can worsen and trigger relapses of their addiction, as shown in Figure 6.2.

Figure 6.2 The common co-occuring relationship between PTSD & addiction: one often triggers the other

PTSD often precedes	**PTSD**	Active addiction often triggers
& triggers addiction	↓ ↑	PTSD symptoms relapse
	Addiction	

Looking back at Figure 6.1 on page 58 above, we can note that addictions and PTSD share a common experience: having a history of repeated childhood and later trauma. Until the effects of the trauma have been addressed head-on over time in a Stage Two full recovery program, it is less likely that the person can achieve any lasting peace.

I have assisted countless patients in their recovery from both addictions and PTSD. When appropriate, I often tell them that they are not mentally ill. Addictions are addictions. While they can mimic "mental illness," contrary to the Bigs' party line, these people are not mentally ill.

Table 6.3 Addictions and PTSD:
Data-based published studies

Date/Author	Sample	PTSD or Addiction	Other findings & Comment
1st Group: [12] **With PTSD** **8 Studies** **1987-98**	24,864+ people, high % with PTSD	For those with PTSD, 1.4-10 x had addictions	High percentage of addictions (as SA/CD) among those with PTSD
2nd Group: [13] **With addictions** **16 Studies** **1986-2007**	4,802 + addicted patients (as CD) & controls	9 to 59% also had PTSD [1.5-12% had PTSD in general population]	These studies probably *underestimate* the percentage of addicted people who also have PTSD Need for routine history for CT/other trauma & screen for PTSD on all addicted
Summary *of above* **24 Studies** **1986-2007**	29,666 people with PTSD or addiction	12-59% SA/CD also had PTSD 1.4-10x CD Odds Ratio SA/CD:PTSD	High association (co-morbidity) between alcoholism/CD and PTSD

Most have PTSD due also to their repeated childhood and later trauma. PTSD is a normal reaction to an abnormal experience. Just as active addiction does, PTSD often mimics mental illness. I suggest that at their first recovery attempt that they focus on the addiction by working a full recovery program for that addiction or problem. After three to six months of successful addiction

---

[12] 1st group compiled from Najavits et al 1997, Ouimette et al 1998; etc
[13] 2nd group compiled from Najavits et al 1997, Saig & Bremner 1999, Langeland et al 2004, Reynolds et al 2005, etc) Other reports support these findings.

recovery, or after the first relapse, I suggest that they begin to address the PTSD in a Stage Two full recovery program, while strengthening treatment for the addiction.

DRUGS DON'T CURE ADDICTIONS

There is no psychiatric or medical drug that cures any addiction or any "mental illness." [25,80,81,83,109] At best, some selected drugs can *assist* in the recovery of some addictions, but these drugs are few, which I will describe in summary form below.

A problem is that today psychiatrists and other physicians are misdiagnosing the emotional and behavioral symptoms of addictions and their almost universal post-trauma effects, including PTSD, as though they are "mental illness" of all sorts. Then they mistreat these people who they misdiagnose with toxic and mostly ineffective psychiatric drugs. They usually neglect to refer the patient to other more effective recovery aids, such as psychotherapy and Twelve Step groups.

In my clinical experience I have found that only six drugs help some people in their recovery from some addictions (Table 6.4). Antabuse (generic name is disulfiram) helps alcoholics not drink by causing a bothersome flu-like reaction if they drink when taking it, while they hopefully work the rest of a full recovery program for alcoholism. Suboxone or Subutex (buprenorphine) is a long-acting opiate that prevents withdrawal for up to 36 hours, yet does not produce the "high," energy, or sedation that other opiates do.

Naltrexone is an opiate antagonist that attaches to the opiate receptors in the brain, thereby blocking the "high" or reinforcing effects of opiates, alcohol and selected other addictions, such as nicotine, pathologic gambling and some eating disorders [156]. Low-dose naltrexone has not been tried in PTSD but may help some of its symptoms such as insomnia; I also recommend it for compulsive overeating and autoimmune illnesses such as multiple sclerosis, Crohn's disease, and the like. Clonidine is an antihypertensive drug that also lessens the severity of opiate withdrawal to a degree. It can also help some people with insomnia sleep better.

BuSpar (buspirone) is safe and effective in reducing fear, anxiety and panic that are common in addictions, PTSD and other "mental illness." It is not addicting and usually has no withdrawal effects. Dilantin (phenytoin) is a safe and effective anti-epilepsy drug that when used for PTSD can help stabilize the brain and nervous system in a subtle way. It may help parts of a trauma- or drug-damaged brain to regenerate, especially in the hippocampus, a brain center for our emotions and memory.

Beyond these drugs, I seldom if ever use conventional psych drugs such as antidepressants, antipsychotics, "mood stabilizers," or benzodiazepines. This is because they are toxic and hurt more than they help people with addictions, PTSD or most "mental illness." These psychiatric drugs commonly cause more problems than they are worth, from direct toxic effects to withdrawal and at worst Drug Stress Trauma Syndrome (Chapter 7, page 67).

Buprenorphine (trade name Suboxone or Subutex) is the only one among these six drugs that is addicting and has a drug (opiate) withdrawal reaction when stopped. But it is clearly a safer, less addicting and more effective choice than methadone long-term.

Any of these drugs used is/are dependent on the person also working a full recovery program for their addiction, including attendance at Alcoholics Anonymous, Narcotics Anonymous, or the like, meetings and working their Twelve Steps long term.

Table 6.4. Selected drugs as aids for alcoholism and other addictions recovery

Drug	*Indications*	*Comment*
Antabuse (disulfiram) [130]	Alcoholism	250 mg by mouth daily. Get sick if drink alcohol. I use it for people who can't stop drinking long term
Suboxone / [130] **Subutex (buprenorphine)**	Opiate dependence	Long acting opiate that prevents withdrawal for up to 36 hours, yet does not produce a "high." Usually superior to methadone programs
Naltrexone [130]	Opiates, alcohol, & other addictions, such as nicotine, pathologic gambling and some eating disorders	Opiate receptor blocker against the "high" or reinforcing effects of opiates, alcohol & these other addictions. Low dose helps other problems/illness.
Clonidine [130]	Opiate withdrawal	Lessens severity of opiate withdrawal. Can also help some people with insomnia. Lowers blood pressure
BuSpar (buspirone) [55,99,131]	Fear, anxiety, panic & depression	Safe & effective in reducing fear, anxiety & panic that are common in addictions, PTSD and other "mental illness."
Dilantin (phenytoin) [29,30,107]	Complex PTSD, Some regular PTSD	Safe anti-epilepsy drug that when used for PTSD can help stabilize the brain & nervous system subtly & may help parts of a trauma- or drug-damaged brain regenerate.

But with the onset of the influence of the "Bigs," especially Big Pharma, Big Government and Big Insurance, physicians (usually as "medical directors" of the addiction treatment program) began to diagnose and treat other "mental illness" than addictions with progressively more psych drugs. Since the early 1990s this practice has overtaken nearly all in-patient and out-patient addiction treatment programs today. I am aware of only one in-patient program that is truly psych drug free (Willingway Hospital in Statesboro, Georgia). I continue to see many of these addicted patients who have bothersome emotional and behavioral symptoms and problems who have been given a string of numerous psych drugs that over time have *not helped* them. Many have suffered numerous painful toxic effects, and most now have or have had in the past one or several debilitating psychiatric drug withdrawal experiences. Many have also gained weight, eaten much junk and processed foods and some are paradoxically malnourished.

In the next chapter I address the final PTSD variant, the Drug Stress Trauma Syndrome, which shows more evidence of how psychiatric drugs are toxic and often traumatic.

7   Drug Stress Trauma Syndrome

HOW PSYCH DRUGS MAY MAKE YOU WORSE

After taking one, and usually more psychiatric drugs, many people end up feeling more distressed. They may experience a worse quality of life than they did before they started taking the drugs. This is what I have come to call the Drug Stress Trauma Syndrome (DSTS), which I describe below. [179] First, let's look at some background information.

ILLEGAL DRUG TOXICITY

We know that illegal drugs often have toxic effects on our body and mind. There are also *legal system* consequences for simple possession and use. If I were to rank ***illegal*** drugs in order of the *most toxic* and dangerous, 1) **phencyclidine** (PCP, "Angel Dust") would be number one. In decreasing order of toxicity, I rank 2) **amphetamines**, including methamphetamine as second; remember that these drugs have the same effects as methylphenidate (Ritalin) and the other stimulant drugs we give 7%, or nearly one in ten of our children every day.

Third, 3) **cocaine**, another stimulant, and other than being shorter acting, not much different than amphetamines. Fourth, is 4) **heroin**, a painkiller like morphine and the other opiates – all with several toxic effects. Fifth are 5) **psychedelic drugs** (erroneously called "hallucinogens"). And finally sixth, 6) **cannabis** (marijuana) is probably the most used illegal drug today, with toxic effects of over-sedation or "dumbing down" (which most *legal* and illegal drugs commonly cause), and lung irritation and damage, dependence/addiction, and withdrawal. Like *all these drugs* their *illegality, way of use* (snorting, smoking or injecting and other use), *lifestyle* adds even more to their toxicity. A recent British study found similar rankings. [119]

As toxic as these six kinds of drugs are, and not to discount their toxicities, to keep it in perspective, the *legal* drugs alcohol and nicotine *disable* and *kill 25 times more* people (about 500,000 yearly deaths) than all of these illegal drugs *combined* (20,000). [49,117]

LEGAL DRUG TOXICITY:
HOW MIGHT PSYCHIATRIC DRUGS MAKE YOU WORSE?

Just because a drug may be legal, i.e., approved by the FDA and readily available from the medical and psychiatric system (physicians, nurses, pharmacists and the like) does not of course, make them any less toxic than the illegal drugs listed above. In fact, some of the legal psychiatric drugs are often *more* toxic, which I describe in Chapters 8 and 9 on page 84 and in Appendix A.1-6 on page 199 . Psychiatrist and psycho-pharmacologist Peter Breggin wrote in 2008, "People commonly use alcohol, marijuana and other non-prescription drugs to dull their feelings. Usually they do not fool themselves into believing they are somehow improving the function of their minds and brains. Yet when people take psychiatric drugs, they almost always do so without realizing that the drugs 'work' by disrupting brain function, that the drugs cause withdrawal effects, and that they frequently result in dangerous and destructive mental reactions and behaviors." [25]

Background Information (this is somewhat technical, so bear with me or skip it for now) In 1999 describing the course of events following any *chronic psychoactive drug-taking* Dr Leo Hollister reviewed Shuster's classic 1961 formulation: 1) the drug perturbs the normal homeostasis of an organ system by virtue of effects on enzymes, neurotransmitters, receptors or second messengers, 2) to compensate, the body responds by increasing the amounts of each. When this occurs the patient may become tolerant to the drug.

3) To maintain the desired effects of the drug, the dose is increased to overcome the body's compensatory reactions. However, increasing doses result in renewed attempts at compensation. 4) Several cycles of this sort may ensue. 5) When a drug is withdrawn, the overcompensated mechanisms are now unopposed, resulting in a withdrawal reaction, generally characterized by symptoms and signs opposite to those usually produced by the drug (physical dependence). [77,143]

Hollister wrote: "This schema was first introduced to explain the sequence of drug-taking of drugs of abuse, which also involve 'psychic [psychological/neurological] dependence.' However, it may be extended to a variety of drugs... It has been long recognized that withdrawal syndromes vary among classes of drug. It 1964, the World Health Organization classified withdrawal syndromes in that fashion: barbiturate-alcohol type, opiate type and stimulant type. *This classification* still applies and *might* be modified now to *include* other drugs not usually abused, but which alter central nervous system function, such as *antidepressants* and *antipsychotics*, where discontinuation syndromes were unanticipated and more subtle and psychic dependence was not [suspected to be] present. We may conclude that any drug which disturbs normal physiology, biochemistry or gene expression may set the stage for such a reaction."(my italics) [77]

Also in 1999 psychiatrist and psycho-pharmacologist David Healy and Richard Tranter described reactions to taking psychiatric drugs, including their withdrawal, as *pharmacological stress diathesis syndromes*. They said, "Recent descriptions of discontinuation syndromes following treatment with antidepressants and antipsychotics, in some cases long lasting, challenge both public and scientific models of addiction and drug dependence. Antipsychotic and antidepressant drug dependencies point to a need to identify predisposing constitutional and personality factors in the patient, pharmacological *risk factors in the drug* and aspects of *therapeutic style* that may contribute to the development of *stress syndromes*. The stress syndromes following antipsychotics also point to the *probable* existence of a *range of syndromes* emerging within treatment. The characteristics of these need to be established." (my italics). [73] Similarly, psycho-pharmacologist Ross Baldessarini and AC Vignera have called these psychiatric drug effects *pharmacologic stress, iatrogenic pharmacologic stress,* and *drug discontinuation-associated stress* [13] —**End** of Background information section

Ranking the legal psychiatric drugs in decreasing order as I did above for the illegal drugs, first are 1) the **antipsychotic** drugs, which are generally so disabling and toxic that they have been shown to cause early death. [25,161,162] Second are 2) the **antidepressant** drugs, which often *cause* an increase in suicidal thoughts and completed suicides, as well as homicides, when compared with placebo pills. [25,80,81] Coming in as a close third are 3) the **stimulants** of the Ritalin and amphetamine type (which are nearly all amphetamines of one sort or another). [23,25,129] Fourth are 4) the **benzodiazepine** sedatives ("benzos") whose main toxicities are over-sedation and emotional numbness (similar to the antipsychotics and antidepressants) and probably having the most painful withdrawal syndrome of all legal and illegal drugs for most people. [25,109] Fifth are 5) the **anti-convulsants**, cleverly called "**mood stabilizers**" for marketing purposes, although they have little to do with mood and they commonly cause numerous toxic effects (see page 205) and an often bothersome withdrawal [25,109,179]. For a summary of these toxic drugs see Table A.1 on page 199. I discuss this ranking further in Chapter 9.

The problem is that these drugs are commonly prescribed to and consumed in multiple brand and generic names by trauma survivors, nearly all of whom are misdiagnosed as having one or another "mental illness." I have seen countless patients over the past 20 years who came to me currently taking—or having taken in the past—from five to twenty psych drugs, none of which had helped them significantly with their original complaints for very long. In fact, many of these people had gotten worse.

Table 7.1 Some characteristics of illegal and legal psychoactive drugs [179]

Illegal drugs

• Overdose from toxic effects on body & mind
    • Organ damage from chronic use
    • "Dumbing-down" effect on mental & social function & self esteem
    • Legal system consequences
    • Most-toxic-drug rank: phencyclidine (PCP), amphetamines, cocaine, heroin, psychedelics, cannabis

Legal drugs – have similar and more toxic effects

• Organ damage from chronic use (e.g., obesity, diabetes, brain/nerve damage)
    • "Dumbing-down" effect on mental & social function & self esteem
    • Forced drugging by Hospital, Court & State system
    • Withdrawal common & bothersome; often harmful to self & others; commonly *misdiagnosed*
    • Akathisia ± withdrawal akathisia → suicide & homicide
    • Violence common with both legal & illegal
    • "Mental illness" labeling → fear & shame, discrimination, isolation
    • Betrayal-trauma by authority figures, may remind of parents

GENESIS OF DRUG STRESS TRAUMA SYNDROME

Over these years of assisting these people, I began to notice a pattern wherein a vicious cycle unfolded. With the above and other information throughout this book, you may be able to see that taking any of these drugs is often unpleasant, usually doesn't work well, and may be detrimental to your current and future mental health. Here is how I have seen that the Drug Stress Trauma Syndrome (DSTS) usually comes about:

The person enters the health care system with one or more psychological or psychiatric symptoms or signs, from bothersome fear, anxiety, to sadness, low energy, to a behavior or relationship problem, or the like. The intake clinician usually does not carefully look for the three most common causes of these symptoms—a recent significant loss, a history of repeated trauma/PTSD and alcohol or other drug dependence. Instead, after a brief (influenced by health insurance or government treatment time limitations) and a cursory evaluation (influenced by the clinician's training and skills), and usually with no physical or laboratory examination, a psychiatric diagnosis is made.

This initial diagnosis may be in error, such as "depression," an "anxiety disorder," "bipolar disorder," "ADHD," a "psychosis," or the like. [87,185] But it satisfies several key people: the health insurance or other authorities' requirements, the clinician, the drug industry, and/or any number of authority figures (boss, court, probation officer, teachers or other school administration, parents or other family members) and, at least temporarily, the patient.

Not addressing the likely trauma effects or the alcohol or other drug effects, a short cut of one or more psych drugs is prescribed. The clinician usually gives the patient no warning about drug toxicity or drug withdrawal, and offers no counseling or psychotherapy. Perhaps unknowingly acting in their favor long term, up to 25% of patients do not get the prescription filled. But for those who start taking the drug(s), the first toxic effect of "medication spellbinding," chemical dissociation or numbing occurs, even though the patient may not be fully aware of it. An unaware observer—trying to be objective—may conclude something like, "So far, so good."

But sooner or later, the patient either stops taking or forgets to take the drug, and for most psych drugs, one of the most common toxic effects begins to occur—drug *withdrawal.* If the withdrawal symptoms are bothersome enough, the patient usually calls or sees their prescribing clinician or physician who should—but usually does not—recognize them as being in drug withdrawal. Instead, they misinterpret the symptoms as a re-emergence or worsening of the patient's original misdiagnosis' symptoms or signs. With this misinterpretation, or second misdiagnosis, they commonly then prescribe a higher drug dose—or a different or stronger drug. They usually give the patient no education or insight on withdrawal symptoms, and again, no serious psychotherapy or counseling.

The now-vicious cycle continues. Over time, the patient may become progressively more dysfunctional in their personal life, their job functioning and/or in their relationships. As part of the DSTS, they often become physically ill, with one or more emergency department visits, medical or psychiatric hospitalizations, arrests, family dysfunction, relationship breakups, and increasing medical costs and debts. Eventually, similar to people with alcohol or drug dependence, they may hit a "bottom."

This phenomenon and process is what I have come to call the Drug Stress Trauma Syndrome, the genesis of which I summarize in Table 7.2. Using definitions of each of the terms, I show a simple summary of DSTS in Table 7.3 at the top of page 75.

How Common is DSTS?

I don't have a reliable answer to this question. I estimate that DSTS is somewhere between uncommon and to a degree common. From my clinical experience, it may occur in at least a distinct minority of 20% or more of people who take psychiatric drugs long-term.

Table 7.2 Drug Stress Trauma Syndrome (DSTS) Genesis by stages of system-induced psychiatric/psychological illness

Actions	Dynamics
First "Diagnosis"	• With no PTSD or Alc & Drug (Chemical Dependence) assessment, wrong diagnosis is made. e.g., "Depression," "Anxiety Disorder," "Bipolar Disorder," "psychosis," "ADHD," etc.
First "Treatment"	• Not addressing trauma or A & D effects; • Psychiatric drug(s) are then given inappropriately • No warning to patient of toxicity, incl. drug withdrawal • No psychotherapy or counseling →"Medication spellbinding" [14]
Patient eventually ***stops or forgets*** to take drug(s)	
Withdrawal Not Diagnosed	• Misinterpret drug withdrawal symptoms/effects as • "re-emergence/worsening" of original misdiagnosed symptoms or signs (see tables in Appendix) or as • another psychiatric disorder
Withdrawal Mistreated	•Mis-prescribes: • Higher drug dose or • Different or stronger drug • No education on withdrawal symptoms • No psychotherapy or counseling →The *Vicious Cycle* Continues
Deterioration	• Person becomes progressively more dysfunctional ± Physically ill, hospitalizations, arrests, family dysfunction/breaks, increased medical costs & DSTS

---

[14] Medication **Spellbinding** = the capacity of psychoactive drugs to blunt the patient's appreciation of drug-induced mental dysfunction and, at times, to encourage a misperception that they are doing better than ever when they are actually doing worse than ever (from Breggin 2006)[186] See also page 210 in the Appendix.

Table 7.3. Drug Stress Trauma Syndrome (DSTS) Summary

Drug - most psychiatric drugs
Stress - the effects of taking & stopping the drug are not only stressful, but distressing & often disruptive to quality of life
Trauma - repeated distress & disruption to quality of life by the drug effects can be & often are traumatic
Syndrome - it has a recognizable pattern of symptoms & signs
For a further definition of "syndrome" see wikipedia.org/wiki/Syndrome

We need observation, research and data-gathering for more reliable figures. For example, in April 2008 I surveyed 25 *clinicians* (social workers, nurses, therapists and counselors—who were 23 women and 2 men) at a one-day workshop that I gave on trauma and recovery to a total of 65 people. Of these 25 people, • 9 (36%; 8 women and 1 man) had taken antidepressant drugs, • 6 (2/3) of whom had been prescribed and taken *more than one* ADP drug. • 7 of the 9 (77%) said they had felt bothersome toxic effects of the drug(s), • 4 (44%) had thus far experienced a disruptive or bothersome withdrawal syndrome, and, • 2 (22% of the 9) said they had clearly become worse long-term than before they began taking the ADPs. [179]

I did not ask them about their taking other psychiatric drugs. I believe that for their use of antipsychotic drugs, stimulants and benzodiazepines the percentage occurrence of DSTS may be more than 22%, and for "mood stabilizers," aka anticonvulsants, and lithium probably less. I discuss and raise several questions regarding these small and preliminary data after the next section.

CHARACTERISTIC OF DSTS

1. The first characteristic of DSTS is the **vicious cycle** now occurring and described under the genesis section above and in Table 7.2. This vicious cycle contains the stressors and resulting distress described among most of the other characteristics below.

2. **Distress from the toxic effects** of the **drug(s).** While these are many and varied, they frequently include several of the following: depression, confusion, difficulty thinking and focusing, insomnia, metabolic–endocrine system disruption, weight gain, easy irritability, relationship disruption, anorgasmia (no orgasms), drug seeking, suicidality, inability to work, and more (see **Tables A.1-6 in the Appendix** on page **199-209**). These are commonly misinterpreted as being a return of the original symptoms and the first erroneous diagnosis.

3. **Withdrawal effects.** These withdrawal effects can be identical to the toxic effects of the drugs *and* to some of the person's original symptoms, including those of their PTSD, making the differential diagnosis difficult. (See page 202-3 for some key ways to differentiate these 3 sometimes difficult diagnostic areas).

4. **Emotional "roller coaster" effects.** The person may be (seemingly, on the surface) relatively peaceful, content, or numb for hours or longer, only to be followed by varying degrees of emotional and behavioral distress, sometimes markedly so. This experience will often be exaggerated by the upper-downer cycle when the person uses alternating uppers or stimulants (such as caffeine, amphetamines, or Ritalin/stimulant-type drugs to wake up, then later, sedatives to try to sleep). [78,149]

5. **Disrupted sleep,** which tends to lead to a painful state of chronic sleep deprivation. A stressor in itself, this sleep

deprivation can then aggravate their acute and chronic stress state. This disrupted sleep is often aggravated by the upper-downer cycle described above. See Chapter 15 on page 185 for details.

6.   **Treatment failure.** The drug or drugs commonly do not consistently help the person's original symptoms. I have seen countless patients who came to me complaining that even after trying numerous and different psychiatric drugs, that they are either no better, or they are worse. I regularly see "depressed" people who have tried antidepressants [such as   Prozac (fluoxetine), Paxil (paroxetine), Zoloft (sertraline), Wellbutrin (bupropion), Effexor (venlafaxine), Celexa (citalopram), Lexapro (escitalopram), Cymbalta, (duloxitine)], and they are no better—or are often worse. Some of them have also tried the more toxic antipsychotics, with no help, and many have additionally tried anti-convulsants ("mood stabilizers"), lithium, other drugs and benzodiazepines—all to no avail. These repeated treatment failures have contributed to their loss of hope that they can ever get better.

As an example, psychiatrist and psycho-pharmacologist David Healy and his colleagues reported the first results of a remarkable study in North Wales on a population that has been stable for over 100 years regarding their numbers, age, cohorts (groups with things in common), ethnic mix and rurality. It showed that since the introduction of the modern psychiatric drugs in psychiatry that there has been a *fifteen*-fold increase in the rate of admissions to psychiatric inpatient hospitals, and a *three*-fold increase in the rate of forced psychiatric hospital admissions. It also showed that people with bipolar disorders have relapsed sooner and more often. This is a remarkable study. Overall, patients with all psychiatric conditions now appear to spend a greater amount of time in a psych hospital than they would have fifty or 100 years ago. These conditions have worsened to these degrees *despite the* *availability* of supposedly effective and claimed prophylactic drug treatments. These findings are incompatible with drug treatments' being effective in practice for a majority of the patients. [74]

Figure 7.1 Drug Stress Trauma Syndrome Components

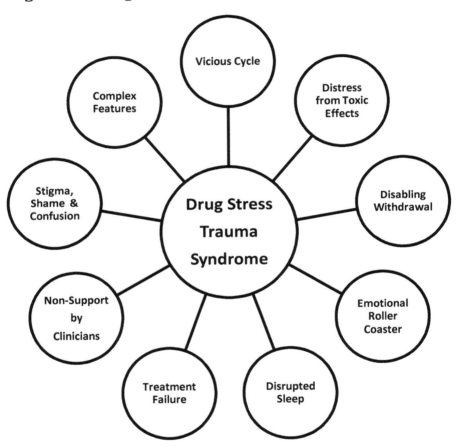

7. **Relative non-support** from psychiatrists, other physicians and clinicians **for using non-drug aids.** Many of my patients have told me of having had this experience, and I have seen it repeatedly in

most dimensions of psychiatry from discussions with colleagues to psychiatry education events.

8. **Stigma, shame and confusion** from and about all of the above, including having been first labeled with a mental illness, promised improvement, and then not getting better with all these "state of the art" psychiatric drugs that they see advertised on TV, in magazines, and elsewhere. These painful feelings also aggravate the above stress responses.

9. The *presence* of DSTS then **reactivates** and often worsens the **underlying PTSD,** alcoholism, other chemical dependence, or other problems in their life. The failure to address and treat the underlying trauma effects is a major factor in the genesis of PTSD. Nearly all of the patients that I saw to have the features of DSTS also had an underlying PTSD. So, rather than psychiatric drugs helping them, a fair percentage of patients with PTSD who are treated with psych drugs appear to be made worse. This drug-mediated worsening, instead of helping their PTSD is likely relatively common among the multi-millions of people who are treated with psychiatric drugs today.

10. *Complex features.* This painful syndrome is *not usually easy to recognize* and diagnose. It usually cannot be readily seen in a 5 to 15 minute medication follow-up check by a physician—which is the usual time approved by the health insurance industry, aka "managed care." If government-run medicine takes hold in the USA, it will get worse. It takes enough time to recognize the many dimensions of DSTS, which usually requires the taking of a careful and thorough initial history from the patient. Then it will likely take a number of follow-up visits and psychotherapy sessions, coordinated with a physician with expertise in treating PTSD and helping people slowly detoxify from psychiatric drugs. Many affected patients won't be able to recognize that it is the drugs that

are making them worse due to their **lack of knowledge** (which this and other books can correct) and the **spellbinding** effects of the drugs (pages 210 through 213 in the Appendix).

HEALING FROM DSTS

For the person who has DSTS or similar symptoms, negotiating their recovery may seem like trying to walk through a mine field. They usually have to deal with multiple people: clinicians, health insurance and payers, family (some of whom may want them to stay "mentally ill"), friends, community, and other authority figures. Navigating all these requires a self-commitment and focus on recovery, with ongoing patience and persistence. Some several thousand traumatized and damaged patients and their families have brought successful lawsuits against the drug makers, especially for **drug-caused** completed **suicides**, **diabetes**, **birth defects** and **addictions**-See Legal summary cites [95] on page 222.

.

Based on my long experience assisting many patients with it, to help someone heal from DSTS the patient and/or clinician usually has to first realize that the patient may have it. If possible, the patient themself may also eventually have to self-diagnose it. The clinician helps them gradually (over months or longer) decrease the dose of the psychiatric drugs and eventually stop taking them. If appropriate, they may also consider referring the patient to a psychotherapist or counselor who knows how to assist with trauma recovery and if indicated, alcohol and other drug dependence recovery. The patient learns to tolerate the emotional and physical pain of withdrawal from the drugs and grieving any trauma effects. They will need to get the right nutrition, attend any appropriate self-help meetings such as AA, NA, ACA, CoDA, EA, or Al-Anon, all while being patient and persistent over months and sometimes years. This is similar to the recovery approach that I have outlined in my other books, including especially *My Recovery* [175]. For more details, see Chapter 15 in Breggin's *Brain Disabling Treatments in Psychiatry* and Chapter 12 on page 141.

QUESTIONS

DSTS has several unknowns and questions. These include: 1) How often does it occur? 2) What is the relationship of DSTS's occurrence to the patient who has a prior history of repeated other kinds of trauma? And 3) how might that affect its occurrence? Thus, 4) How common is DSTS among people with prior PTSD?

Figure 7.2 shows a 2-by-2 chart or two-dimensional model of psychiatric drug exposure and prior repeated trauma as factors in the genesis of DSTS that explores their relationship in 4 possible quadrants. As shown in both upper quadrants, the more prior repeated trauma in a patient will be more likely associated with increased symptoms and signs of mental illness as I summarize in Table 1.2 and in *The Truth about Depression* and *The Truth about Mental Illness*. Likewise, the more people with these symptoms and signs come to clinicians with them, given today's worldview about mental health, the more likely they will be prescribed psychiatric drugs. Given a premise of this chapter, those who get the most psychiatric drugs for the longest time will be the most likely to develop DSTS. By contrast, those in the left lower quadrant will be the least likely to develop DSTS because of their lower exposure to *both* repeated trauma and long-term psychiatric drug use. Finally, in the right lower quadrant of the figure my best medical estimation is that we will need more research and data on those in this category due to the small amount of preliminary data above.

Also 5) How does the distress and trauma of experiencing DSTS affect the PTSD after their trauma in that this may now be their *fourth* trauma? Their 1st original trauma was that which caused the

PTSD. The 2nd occurred when the trauma survivor tried to tell their experience of the trauma to those they thought were supposed to be protecting them, but it was invalidated or rejected by their parents, parent figures or clinicians. The 3rd trauma was

Figure 7.2 Psychiatric Drug Exposure and Trauma

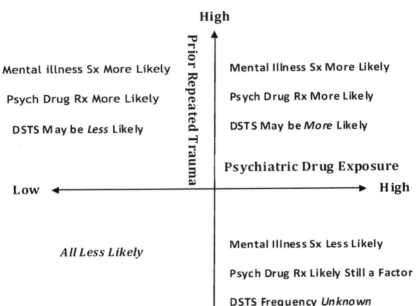

having been labeled as being "mentally ill" when instead they were grieving a significant loss, had PTSD or complex PTSD, or an active addiction. The 4th trauma is their now experiencing the distress of DSTS, including their confusion about the nature and unanswered fact that the psychiatric drugs have not only *not helped* them, but *made them worse* in the form of DSTS.

Problems of denial by physicians and other helping professionals regarding this finding are likely, such as: 1) the possible causal relationship between trauma and subsequent mental illness and 2) the possibility of the reality of DSTS among their patients who not only don't get better but get worse on psychiatric drugs. My experience is that based on their beliefs, most physicians and other helping professionals deny both of these, promoting more toxic drug exposure.

In the next Chapter I begin to describe in some elementary and at times advanced detail the nature of the toxicity of psychiatric drugs, much of which is not mentioned in conventional medical, psychiatric and nursing textbooks, journal articles, and related websites. After that, I go into it in more depth in Chapter 9.

Sidebar: Further comments on the *DSM* Herb Kutchins and Stuart Kirk wrote: "*DSM* is a book of tentatively assembled agreements. [summary = **tentative agreements**] Agreements don't always make sense, nor do they always reflect reality. You can have agreements among experts without validity. Even if you could find four people who agreed that the earth is flat, that the moon is made of green cheese, that smoking cigarettes poses no health risks, or that politicians are never corrupt, such agreements do not establish truth." **From The UK's *Guardian*:** For any statement to be valid there has to be evidence for that statement outside of the statement itself. Thus any textbook of physical disorders will list not just the symptoms of each illness but evidence that exists separate from those symptoms and that is derived from a wide variety of tests. Apart from the disorders listed in the *DSM* as the result of brain trauma, there are no physical tests for any of the disorders listed in the *DSM*. No physical cause has been found for any of these mental disorders. The diagnosis you receive from a psychiatrist is no more than the psychiatrist's opinion of what you have told him. Go to another psychiatrist and you're likely to get a different diagnosis. ... When we keep making a mess of our life we need someone to help us face the truths about which we've been lying to ourselves. But when we are given a diagnosis we disappear behind that diagnosis, and the diagnosis is all the unthinking people see. Dorothy Rowe (2010) Mental health diagnoses mask the real problems - A textbook of mental health disorders makes it far too easy for doctors to label patients–and disregard the roots of suffering. Website is guardian.co.uk, 29 July. For more on *DSM* see pages 12,17,43,111,179,213. This is because a basis for labeling people as "mentally ill" is in the *DSM* and ICD9.

8   Drug Toxicity

Drug toxicity means that a drug's actions and effects are likely to decrease the health and function of our body, mind, and spirit. It is the degree to which a substance is able to harm an exposed person. Most psychiatric drugs are toxic in several ways. Toxicity due to psych drugs covers a spectrum from weight gain and diabetes to mental and emotional blunting to anorgasmia to debilitating withdrawal (Fig 14.1 on page 182). Most toxicity is dose dependent. Drug toxicity is often reflected in a decrease in our function and quality of life. In this chapter and the next I will describe the essence of this toxicity.

Many psychiatrists and other physicians and clinicians *do not warn* their patients—also called "informed consent"—of these likely problems from taking psychiatric drugs. [25,80,81,109,183] Instead, when we go to one of them for help, they are more likely to focus mostly on the benefits of taking the drugs they prescribe.

This chapter includes half of my summary of what mental health consumers and their clinicians can consider as experienced and cutting edge "out of the box" thinking and information on psychiatric drugs. If it gets too ponderous for you, consider moving to the next chapter which continues and expands it in other ways.

CLASSIFYING AND UNDERSTANDING PSYCHIATRIC DRUGS

No classification of psychiatric drugs is easy or adequate to explain what they actually do and don't do. I will describe two such ways of sorting out the *actions* of these drugs. Even though these ways may be confusing, they can begin to show us how **non-specific** in action and **toxic** these drugs can be and are and how *imperfect* any seemingly simple classification can be.

The Usual Drug Classification is Not Accurate

The most common way of describing psychiatric drugs is to classify them by their *presumed* main actions: antipsychotics, antidepressants, sedatives, "mood stabilizers," and stimulants. But there are three problems with using this kind of categorization:

> 1) It is not accurate, and
> 2) The drugs do not work well for each named action, and
> 3) They are generally more toxic then helpful.

Antipsychotic drugs are *not specific* for treating or curing psychosis.* They work by *disabling* the *brain* and *body* to such an extent that the person is so sedated, slowed, dulled, and dampened in their ability to think and respond and numbed in their feelings that they are unable to interact with themselves and others in a healthy way. Family, friends, and others commonly observe them as being "better" because they stop "acting out" or expressing their pain, and through the action of the drug the person believes they are better (see pages 210-213 and Table A.7 on page 211). But they are nearly always actually **not** better and are often worse.

Three example, independent studies on the antipsychotic drug risperidone (Risperdal—reminder: most all drug names are made up for marketing purposes) illustrate some of the ways that it—and other antipsychotics—effect us (Table 8.1). These 3 carefully-conducted studies showed that risperdone causes such an extensive *decrease* in the *metabolism* of the brain's mental and emotional centers that the person taking it can't share their real thoughts and feelings. This profound blockage of neuro-transmission causes apathy and indifference, also called a *chemical lobotomy*.[25,26,91,100,116]

* I explain more about the nonspecific and "shotgun" actions of most psychiatric drugs in Chapter 14 on pages 181-4. Read that short section now if you have time and interest. Also see Figure 14.1 on p.182.

Table 8.1. Risperidone (Risperdal) toxicity –3 example studies [25]

Research Reports	Study details	Findings
Liddle et al 2000 11 schizophrenic patients had PET scans of brain (frontal cortex, thalamus, ventral striatum) [100]	• 1 dose risperidone → Decreased metabolism of mental & emotional centers • 6 weeks risperidone → • Extensive decrease in metabolism of mental & emotional centers. No longer communicating their symptoms	Profound blockage of neurotransmission, causing apathy & indifference, also called *chemical lobotomy* (Breggin 2008)
Ngan et al 2002 PET scans of brain (frontal cortex, thalamus, ventral striatum) [116]	• Reproduced same findings. • Called it deactivation. • Said healthy control group was needed (see below Lane et al).	These brain disabling effects are due to the drug, not schizophrenia
Lane et al 2004 PET scans of brain (frontal cortex, thalamus, ventral striatum) in **9 healthy volunteers** [91]	• 1 2-mg dose risperidone → Decreased metabolism of mental & emotional centers • 6 weeks risperidone → • Extensive decrease in metabolism of mental & emotional centers. No longer communicating their symptoms	Thus, these brain disabling findings are due to the drug, not schizophrenia. Proof of high toxicity to normals
Summary **3 independent studies**	• Risperidone causes an **extensive decrease** of **metabolism** of mental & emotional centers	These **brain disabling** effects are due to the drug, **not** schizophrenia/other disorder. All other antipsychotics do the same [25,26]

Antidepressant drugs also are *not specific* for treating or curing depression. They act in several ways, including by sedating similar to the effects of antipsychotics, and/or by stimulating. They also cause varying degrees of psychological and emotional numbing. [25]

Sedative drugs - By contrast, sedative drugs are usually more specific by decreasing fear and anxiety. By far the most prescribed sedatives are the benzodiazepines. Their problem is that they also act in a "shotgun" fashion in that they tend to numb all of our feelings and emotions, not just fear and anxiety. More on them below and in the next chapter. [49,83,130]

"Mood stabilizers" are actually expensive anticonvulsants with moderate to strong *sedative* effects. They are not otherwise specific for treating any other disorder than epilepsy, and they are toxic (Table 8.2). The term "mood stabilizers" is a contrived marketing device to sell these drugs. It is a buzz word that has no other meaning in medicine or pharmacology. [25,109,110]

Lithium, similar to lead and mercury, is a toxic metal with sedating properties that has *no beneficial use* in medicine or psychiatry. Its effects are also not specific for manic depressive or "bipolar" disorder or any other illness or condition. [109,110]

Stimulants are an accurate term to describe their actions. They are strong stimulants of our brain and body, including our cardiovascular system [83,130]. But like all the other psychiatric drugs, they are *non-specific* for treating any disorder or condition, including "ADHD" and "ADD," and they are toxic (Table 8.2).

> Note: When referring to all these drugs I will use the terms psychiatric, psychoactive, and psych interchangeably.

Table 8.2. Toxicity and Efficacy of Psychiatric Drugs

Toxicity → Drug Type ↓	Numbing Mental & Emotional	Suicidality Increased	Akathisia, Over-Stimulation	Weight Gain, Diabetes	Other Physical Toxicity	Withdrawal Severity	Efficacy
Anti-Psychotics	+++ - ++++	+ - +++	+ - +++	+++ - ++++	++ - ++++ *	++ - +++	Worsen course chronically
Anti-Depressants	++ - ++++	+ - ++ [2-3x**]	+ - +++	+ - +++	++	+ - ++++	2-8% > placebo; often worsen chronically
Benzo-diazepines	+ - +++	+ ?	No data	+ ?	No data	+ - ++++	Effective for acute anxiety; > 1 wk highly addicting
"Mood Stabilizers"	+ - ++	+ - ++	+	+ - ++	+	+ - ++	A buzz word. Not specific
Lithium	+ - +++	Conflicting data	±	+ - +++	++ - ++++	+ - ++	Toxic. Not specific for any disorder
Stimulants	A false, chemical upper	No data; may be ↑ in some	++ - ++++	—	+ - +++	+ - +++	Marginal to worsen to severe

* Esp. *Movement* disorders ** Most often via akathisia Key: + = Some toxic effect (v. normalcy), ++ = moderately toxic, +++ = advanced toxicity, ++++ = severe toxicity

THE DRUGS DON'T WORK WELL

None of the commonly used psychiatric drugs works well to lessen the symptoms of any "mental illness" *long term*, as Moncrieff describes in her book *The Myth of the Chemical Cure* and as I summarize in the right hand column of Table 8.2 above and in more detail in my two books *The Truth about Depression* and *The Truth about Mental Illness*. However, here are a few psych drugs that are relatively non toxic and more specific in their action.

Buspirone (BuSpar) is a non-shotgun and usually non-sedating drug that is more specific long-term for *fear* and *anxiety* and is also successfully *antidepressant* in effect. It is among the least toxic and safest of all the psych drugs, and it has little or no withdrawal effects. This is in contrast to most of the other psychiatric drugs, which are toxic and have bothersome withdrawal syndromes. In summary it tends to work successfully long-term to lessen fear, anxiety and panic, as well as for "depression." [55,99,131]

Phenytoin (Dilantin) is a relatively safe and nontoxic inexpensive anticonvulsant with essentially no sedative properties that I and some other physicians use for selected people with PTSD. It is a tried-and-true drug that has been used effectively to treat epilepsy since 1938. It acts by reducing electrical conductance among brain cells by stabilizing neurons without impairing normal brain function—unfortunately which most of the newer anticonvulsants do. There is some evidence that it helps the often trauma-shrunken hippocampus return to a normal size and heal in people with PTSD. [29,30] Aside from treating and preventing seizures, it is also an option to use in the treatment of trigeminal neuralgia and for certain cardiac arrhythmias. I have found it to work well in concert with buspirone as part of a full recovery program for people with PTSD. [29,30,107]

Benzodiazepine and **barbiturate sedatives** *work well* ***short term*** only in the treatment of fear and anxiety associated with **medical** and **surgical procedures** and in some psychiatric **emergencies** such as intense and debilitating fear and anxiety that are unresponsive to talk-downs. They are useful in these situations for a few days to a week maximum, but have a gradually to rapidly increasing tolerance and thus begin to lose their effectiveness longer term, and are ***highly addicting***, especially benzodiazepines. Benzodiazepines have one of the most debilitating withdrawal reactions in all of medicine.

Otherwise most psychiatric drugs don't work well and their shotgun effects (page 182) and moderate to high toxicity argues against using them, as numerous psychiatrists and those who have studied them have carefully observed. [25,80,81,49,130]

MORE TOXIC THAN HELPFUL

I summarize the toxicity of psychiatric drugs in a series of tables starting in this chapter and elsewhere in this book, including the Appendix, i.e., **Tables A.1 - A.7** (page **199**). In Table 8.2 on page 88 above I estimate the degree of toxicity for each drug category regarding six common and bothersome areas. These include: mental and emotional numbing, increased suicidality, akathisia or over-stimulation, weight gain, diabetes, other physical toxicity, and withdrawal severity. Left off this list in Table 8.2 is anorgasmia (can't have orgasms) and decreased libido (sexual desire).

These estimates are based on my long clinical experience and my reading of the psychiatric and medical literature from the 1970s to the present, including especially that of widely respected and published psychiatrists Joanna Moncrieff, Peter Breggin, Grace Jackson, Joseph Glenmullin, David Healy, J. Douglas Bremner, and others listed in the reference section at the end of this book.

90

I have observed that most physicians and psychiatrists (and most non-physician clinicians) who recommend psychiatric drugs to their patients and clients are not fully aware of the degree of their toxicity. They tend to recommend and prescribe them without clear explanations or warnings—or obtaining written informed consent—regarding how toxic these drugs are and how unlikely it will be for them to get positive results long term. They also **do not usually *warn*** their patients *about the common and often severe withdrawal reaction* that most suffer *when they miss one or more doses* or if they try to *stop* or even *taper the dose.* 80 I found only one study from 1997 that evaluated this problem. In it researchers Young and Currie said "...a sizable minority about 1/3 of physicians *denied* being confidently *aware* of the existence of antidepressant *withdrawal* symptoms. Education about discontinuation [withdrawal] reactions, including the hallmark features, symptoms, and course, is needed for both psychiatrists and family practice physicians." 183 [my italics]

Table 8.3 Psychiatrist and GP Knowledge of Antidepressant Withdrawal (WD) in 1997 183

Knowledge & Skill	*Psychiatrist (n = 50) %*	*GP* (n = 53) %*
Confident awareness of Antidepressant WD	72 yes / **28 no = Lack of knowledge**	30 yes / **70 no**
Direct experience treating patients with WD	*66 yes* / **34 no**	42 yes / **58 no**
Advise patients about WD effects (symptoms)	10 yes (20%) / **40 (80%) no**	9 yes (17%) / **44 no (83%)**

Authors' conclusion: "Antidepressant discontinuation reactions are preventable and simple to treat" *GP = General Practice physician

I have had countless patients come for help because their psych drugs —often a string of *multiple* drugs over time—have *not helped* them or had *made them worse* than they were before they started taking them. [179] Many had not been able to stop taking the drugs due to having experienced a difficult to severe withdrawal. Usually they had *not been warned* about their toxicity, withdrawal, and the likelihood that the drug would not work. [80] Many had gained weight (of from 10 to 140 pounds), had lost their ability to have orgasms, and had bothersome insomnia, mental and emotional dulling and most had experienced painful withdrawals. [25,81] Many physicians prescribe more drugs to try to treat the toxic effects or withdrawal, and tell them their symptoms are due to their original disorder or another one, the most common recent one being "bipolar disorder."

A SIMPLER CLASSIFICATION

The second way of sorting out and understanding psychiatric drugs may be simpler, although I will show how it also has contradictions. This classification says that there are three main kinds of psychoactive drugs: **uppers**, **downers**, and "**all arounders.**" [78,149] Other terms for these three categories are stimulants, sedatives, and psychedelics ("mind-altering or mind-expanding"). In psychiatry and medicine today the first two of these drug types are by far the most commonly prescribed, as I list in Table 8.2 above. A problem is that in sorting out which of these effects a given drug or drug type will bring in an individual person —which can be unpredictable and confusing. [25,187]

Many in these psych drug categories have dual actions. For example, the original or "first generation" (1970 to about 1988) **antidepressants** were mostly *sedating* (i.e., "antianxiety" – here remember that 4 of 5 "depressed" people have bothersome anxiety[173]), but also often cause a concomitant painful *stimulating* effect or triggering more fear/anxiety. [25] By contrast, the newer antidepressants are mostly stimulating, but can also often cause a disabling sedative effect. [25] For example, I have seen many who took paroxetine (Paxil) to have been over stimulated, and others who took the same drug in the same doses who were over sedated.

Antipsychotics are mostly **sedating**, but like the older antidepressants they often cause a concomitant bothersome stimulant effect or anxiety, the most extreme manifestation of which is called *akathisia*. [173] The conclusion is that **neither drug type's action is specific to its name**. "Antidepressants" and "antipsychotics" are actually "shotgun" type drugs. They do not usually hit a specific target such as "depression" or "psychosis." Instead, they hit a **combination** of our • anxiety, • thinking and deciding ability, • sexual functioning, • brain and • body metabolism, • often promote violence and • other aspects of our life negatively (Figure 14.1 p. 182. These could thereby fit under the "all arounder" category, but without any mind expansion.

By contrast, **downer** or sedative drugs such as alcohol, barbiturates, and benzodiazepines function by mostly sedating us. And **upper** drugs such as nicotine, caffeine, cocaine, and the amphetamines function mostly by stimulating us. [130,187]

Opiate pain killers may act as downers and sedate us. But many people use them recreationally because they also give them energy and motivation to work and interact with people, thereby making them appear to be antidepressant in action. [130,187]

Cannabis (marijuana) effects are mostly sedating, but many use them for their mild psychedelic or mind expanding effects, which can temporarily lift the spirit, even though at high doses it dampens other mental functions such as short-term and working memory. Cannabis is also one of the most effective anti-nausea drugs known, which is in part why some 21 states now have provisions for its use in some medical conditions, aka medical marijuana.

Important in the above is the long-held truism called "**set** and **setting**." A drug's effect may be influenced by the user's mindset combined with their social setting. [160] For example, drinking the downer drug alcohol at a party or social situation can seem to stimulate us by disinhibiting or releasing our inhibitions. But drinking alcohol when we are alone and low in energy will more likely sedate us, and when we are already feeling sad it may help or trigger us to cry.

THE DRUGS *CAUSE* PSYCHIATRIC SYMPTOMS

Some of my patients have reported that they felt better *for a time* while taking psychiatric drugs, but that the drugs then stopped working or they got worse (the extreme of which I call Drug Stress Trauma Syndrome, described in Chapter 7 on page 67 above). It has been my long clinical experience that the **three most common causes** of **psychiatric and psychological symptoms** (emotional and behavioral pain) today are:

1) Unhealed **effects** of **repeated trauma**,

2) Difficulty handling conflict, grieving significant losses [147] and **other unhealed core issues** [188], including ego inflation, that are common among trauma survivors, and

3) **Psychiatric** (and sometimes other medical) **drug toxicity**, including drug **withdrawal** [25].

Psychiatric symptoms do not usually appear spontaneously. Too many clinicians are unaware of these 3 common causes. Instead, they have bought into the claims of the Bigs (Pharma, Gov,

Psychiatry, Academia and Insurance) that these symptoms and signs are due to a genetically transmitted disorder of brain chemistry for which the only effective treatment is psychiatric drugs, and in the extreme, electroconvulsive treatment (ECT). As numerous observant psychiatrists, psychologists, and other observers have pointed out over the last 200 years, there have been **no proven biological causes** *for any common mental disorder or illness*, including genetic transmission and bad brain chemistry.
109,132,173,174

Most clinicians *do not carefully screen for* a trauma history or for PTSD. Many to most of them do not consider whether the ***drugs may be causing the person's symptoms*** – either by direct toxicity or withdrawal from the drug. I summarize these symptoms, signs and withdrawal manifestations for each drug category in Tables A.1 through A.7 from pages 199 through 209 in the Appendix.

The adverse effects of antidepressants and antipsychotics are not confined to psychiatric patients. They are also often used "off label" (not FDA-approved) as anti-anxiety drugs and sedatives, and the antipsychotics for their antiemetic (anti-nausea) properties, to control hiccups, to treat migraine headaches, as antidotes for drug-induced psychosis, and sometimes to strengthen the effects of opiate painkillers. Thus any of the adverse effects of these toxic drugs may occur in these settings outside of usual psychiatry.

In some cases, it can be difficult to determine if the adverse drug effect is caused by direct drug toxicity, by drug withdrawal, or by both.

Take a few minutes to look carefully at the **Tables** in this chapter and in the **Appendix** (Tables **A.1-6** on pages **199-209**) regarding the toxic effects of psychiatric drugs.

* Study them carefully if you have time or interest.

95

Have you or anyone you know experienced any of these symptoms or behaviors? Has anyone you may have worked with or seen described on TV or in other media experienced any of these? If you are a clinician, have any of your patients or clients experienced any of these? If your answer is yes, then the *drug* or its *withdrawal* after stopping it or missing a dose may be causing your symptom, behavior or problem, and, once again, you may not be mentally ill.

I repeat: **You may not be mentally ill.** But most clinicians won't likely know this crucial information.

If you wish, you can look for a helping professional with expertise in this area of psychiatric drug toxicity, withdrawal and what to do about it. It may be *hard to find* such a specialist. If you find them, see them for an evaluation. If they say that you have a mental illness (other than PTSD, which is not a mental illness—though its symptoms can simulate one—but it is only a normal reaction to an abnormal and distressing event or series of such events) and if they try to give you more drugs, find a second or third helping professional for their opinion.

Because of the continued misinformation about psychiatric drugs that is circulated and promoted on TV, the print media, and by the Bigs, I will go deeper and discuss it from still other angles in the next chapter.

A Note on taking antipsychotic drugs long-term compared with smoking cigarettes:

Cigarette smokers die 15 to 20 years earlier than non-smokers.

Those who take anti-psychotics long-term die 25 years earlier than those who don't; this has less to do with lifestyle than the toxicity of the drug itself. [161, 162]

9   Part 2 - Psychiatric Drug Toxicity in Perspective

I n this chapter I continue and expand the previous two by describing the toxicity of psychiatric drugs from the perspective of a *spectrum* that spans from the most to the least toxic among them, though now in some more detail. This may be useful information for all who *have taken* them, take them *now*, or may be *offered* any of these drugs in the *future*. Bear with me if this seems too repetitive, or go to the next section or chapter.

Others and I define toxicity as the *degree to which a substance is able to* decrease or stifle the health and function of our body, mind, and spirit. BigPharma prefers to disguise and minimize these toxic effects by calling them "side effects." To help understand the toxicity of most psychiatric drugs, I have below put them in perspective, ranking them from the *most* to the *least* toxic (see Table 9.1). Comparing them to the most toxic of drugs used in medicine—*anticancer drugs* (cancer chemotherapy) which kill most body cells if we continue taking them beyond what is recommended, and potent *anesthetics* used in surgery that require a full-time rescue physician anesthesiologist or nurse anesthetist just to keep us breathing and alive—we can see that the commonly used psychiatric drugs are not far behind them in their degree of toxicity. The most toxic of these are the antipsychotics.

ANTIPSYCHOTIC DRUGS

Antipsychotics are the most toxic of all the psychiatric drugs (see Table 9.1 below and Tables A.1 and A.2 on pages 199 to 209 in the Appendix). Called legal "slow poison" by some experts, they shorten our life span by about 25 years when we take them long term. [25,161,162] They are also called major tranquilizers and

Table 9.1 Psychiatric Drug Toxicity in Perspective

Drug Type	Toxicity Severity	Description	GAF[15]	Withdrawal
Anti-Cancer drugs	10	Kills nearly all body cells, & person if they continue taking	Low	Most normal cells regenerate when stop
Surgical Anesthesia	9	Puts us in a "coma" beyond sleep. Total incapacitation during surgery.	0 - 2	Takes **hours** to awaken fully
Antipsychotics	8	Mental/emotional numbing; disrupt body metabolism & health; *shortened life span* for APs	1 - 40	Commonly severe & long
Antidepressants	7			
Stimulants [16] - incl. nicotine	6	Over-stimulate, arterial narrowing, emotional disruption, insomnia	40 - 70	May be severe & long
Benzodiazepine sedatives	5	Emotional & some mental numbing		Commonly severe & long
Antiepileptics incl. lithium[17]	4	Sedating, esp. early. High toxicity.	Dep- ends on several factors [18]	Mild to moderate
Opiates[19]	2-3	Varies: have antidepressant effects, energize, &/or sedate		Up to 2 weeks long
Buspirone	1	Anti fear, subtle antidepressant		None usually
Drug-free life	0	Healthier	70 - 100	None

---

[15] GAF = Global Assessment of Functioning usually *from the drug alone's toxicity*

[16] Addictive lifestyle & illegality can worsen functioning & health

[17] Marketing term for these = "mood stabilizers"

[18] Degree of repeated childhood trauma, (mis)diagnosis & (mis)treatment, & lack of a full recovery program.

neuroleptics (a short term that emphasizes how they *seize* [leptic = Greek for seize/seizure] our brain and nervous system to produce a state of apathy, lack of initiative, limited range of emotion, and commonly cause neurological damage similar to Parkinson's disease when taken longer than a few days).

For people with chronic psychotic symptoms, antipsychotic drugs act mostly by sedating and numbing their mental and emotional abilities and functioning that they become so numb and "dumbed down" that they are unable to express themselves spontaneously. These inhibiting effects include dampening the ways people spontaneously and constructively previously expressed themselves *and* behaved and ways that bothered them and those around them, including especially their family or other close people. Abbreviated: chemical brain/mind straight-jackets.

Antipsychotics are among the most difficult of all the psychiatric drugs to stop due to at least two factors:

1) Painful and long-term withdrawal symptoms when they miss taking a dose or when they may try to stop them, and

2) Forced drugging of the person by clinicians, the courts, and families, often a subtle to hidden phenomenon.

Most of the *families* of people with chronic psychotic symptoms have not only *supported* drugging their family member by clinicians and often by the courts, but they have played a major role in *forcing* the person to take antipsychotics over time. The families are not all to blame, since they have not usually been told the truth. Information and facts have been available for decades which show that people with schizophrenia do better over time with psycho-social support and kindness, specific psychotherapy long term (as psychologist Bert Karon[84] and others describe [154]), and **avoiding** psychiatric drugs, especially antipsychotics. [25,181,182]

Yet these groups (clinicians, courts, and usually families) have declined these more long-term effective treatment and recovery methods for their patients and family members, and instead have chosen to subdue and control them with drugs. Families do have to set appropriate boundaries and limits when their "psychotic" relative acts-out inappropriately, but they can do so without effectively restraining them with toxic drugs. [84,157,174]

The evidence is strong that people with schizophrenia have a significant childhood and later trauma history, which others and I have summarized. [128,174] A problem is that the family and "mental health" *system* from which the person comes is itself usually not fully aware of this important information, and being therapeutically *dysfunctional,* they are not usually open to using it.

An increasingly large group of people who are prescribed antipsychotics include those *without* chronic psychotic symptoms. Because they tend to be more functional than those with psychosis, there is seldom pressure on them from the courts, although their clinicians and family usually still encourage them to keep taking the antipsychotic(s). But once they start taking them, the antipsychotics' bothersome withdrawal usually forces many to continue taking them long term—and usually to their detriment.

Perhaps the most disturbing group of people who are prescribed these dangerous antipsychotic drugs are children, which I discuss in the next chapter.

ANTIDEPRESSANTS

While not quite as toxic as antipsychotics, antidepressants still have a sizable downside. A related and telling fact is that drug companies still get countless law suits almost daily from people who have been injured by antidepressant drugs (see Table A.10 in the Appendix on page 222. Similar to antipsychotics, antidepressants cause a range of mental, emotional and physical discomforts and problems, as shown in Tables 8.2 and 9.1 above and A.1-2 on pages 199-202 in the Appendix. These two detailed tables show how similar antidepressants are to antipsychotics in their detrimental effects on our mind, emotions and body .

I wrote in my book *The Truth about Depression*, "The truth about depression is that it is not as advertised. It is not what some special-interest groups tell us. It is not the single, simple disorder that drug companies and some mental health groups may claim. It is not simply a genetically transmitted disorder of brain chemistry. It is not a brain serotonin problem. And it *does not reliably respond to antidepressant drugs*. And these drugs are *not the only available recovery aid*." (italics added) [173]

In that book I reviewed several reasons why antidepressant drugs (ADPs) don't work adequately for most people with depression. The success rate for ADP drugs ranges *at best* from 1/3 (common) to 2/3 (less common) of all depressed people who take them, although that success is too often short-lived. This means that for the other 1/3 to 2/3 of people, ADP drugs don't work sufficiently well for them, if at all. Some of the reasons for their low success rates include the following clinical and political observations and concerns.

1) Antidepressant drugs are not specific for treating depression. They have a "shotgun" effect whereby other symptoms and neural systems are negatively affected, as mentioned above (Figure 14.1 on page 182).

2) Like most other psychiatric drugs, ADPs have a high number and frequency of *toxic effects*, which the drug industry has downplayed for decades by calling them "side effects."

3) Of those patients who are prescribed ADPs, 30% never get their prescription filled, and of those who do, another 40% stop taking the drug within from one to three months—primarily due to these toxic effects, such as weight gain, anorgasmia, over-sedation or over-stimulation. [126] Antipsychotics and "mood stabilizers" have similar drawbacks. [25]

4) Drug companies tend to exaggerate the successes of ADPs and their other psychiatric drugs. Of course, the drugs that they promote are those for which they still hold the patent for exclusive rights to market and sell [173]. Drug companies seldom market drugs for which they no longer hold a patent.

While antipsychotic drugs are more toxic than antidepressants, some antidepressants are more difficult to taper and stop than others. In my clinical experience assisting people in this process, the most difficult antidepressants to stop have been Effexor (trade name venlafaxine) and Paxil (paroxetine), for which a slower taper over a much longer time than usual is commonly needed. The next most difficult to taper is Zoloft (sertraline), and the other antidepressants vary in their difficulty to stop.

In summary, antidepressant drugs are not specific for treating depression, do not work well, have a high incidence of bothersome toxic effects, are usually expensive and once started they are painfully difficult to stop taking [173].

STIMULANTS

Stimulant drugs include amphetamines (with various trade names), methylphenidate (Ritalin), cocaine, caffeine, nicotine, and some miscellaneous drugs. Until the promotion of their use for ADHD, they had few indications in medicine. In reality they still do.

Charles L. Whitfield, M.D.

It is strange that the same amphetamine/methylphenidate stimulants, including "crystal methamphetamine" that are sold on the street illegally as a part of the drug culture for which countless people are arrested daily, are also prescribed in doctor's offices and clinics and given daily by parents and school nurses as a legitimate treatment for "ADHD" and "ADD." Ritalin has a similar structure as crystal methamphetamine and an essentially identical effect on the nervous system and body, yet we give this toxic drug to some 8 million of our children at least twice almost every day of the week. What makes "crystal meth" somewhat more toxic is their contaminants and the lifestyle it can take to make and get them. [130]

In a 1976 controlled trial of Ritalin versus placebo in children, researchers observed that: "[The children became] distinctly more bland or 'flat' emotionally, lacking both the age-typical variety and frequency of emotional expression. They responded less, exhibited little or no initiative and spontaneity, offered little indication of either interest or aversion, showed virtually no curiosity, surprise or pleasure, and seemed devoid of humor. Jocular comments and humorous situations passed unnoticed. In short, while on active drug treatment the children were relatively but unmistakably affectless, humorless, and apathetic." [129] Influenced by the Bigs, these strong negative results have been mostly ignored by the mainstream and clinical media. [174] This is once again a sad reflection on our unaware and mostly dysfunctional mental health system—in the USA and worldwide.

I summarize the toxic effects of these drugs in the second and third left hand columns of Table 9.1 above. Similar to most psychiatric drugs, once these stimulants are taken regularly over time they are hard to stop. Also similar to taking most psychiatric drugs, it usually takes great motivation to taper and stop them—even while seeing a *skilled clinician* who is *fully aware* of how to so *assist them*—as they taper and finally stop.

Benzodiazepine Sedatives

Benzodiazepines have been the most commonly prescribed sedating, anti-anxiety, and hypnotic (for sleep) sedative drugs for the past few decades. For 25 years—from 1960 when available until the mid-1980s—the makers of benzodiazepines and many psychiatrists denied that these drugs were addicting. (As a full time faculty member in a medical school department of psychiatry for 8 years, I saw and heard my fellow faculty deny that benzos were addicting.) After some 30 years after they were put on the market authorities reluctantly and only partially admitted this aspect of their toxicity. Even so, these over-20 benzo chemical clones of one another are still prescribed as though they are not among the most addicting of all psychoactive drugs, much less that they also numb the mind, feelings, body and spirit.

Even so, benzodiazepines are the safest and most effective anti-fear and anxiety drugs for *acute* medical emergencies such as heart attacks and the like, and surgical procedures, when needed and prescribed for a few days only. [83,187] But when they are taken for longer than that, they become progressively less effective, more toxic, numbing and highly addicting. [49,130]

In my decades of clinical experience, benzodiazepines are perhaps the most difficult to taper and stop of all the psychiatric drugs for most people. The faster acting and short half-life benzodiazepines such as alprazolam (trade name Xanax) and lorazepam (Ativan) are usually more difficult to taper and stop than the longer acting benzodiazepines. This observation forms the basis and rationale for transferring to a long half-life benzodiazepine such as diazepam (Valium). [49] I show the half-life and equivalent doses of many of the benzodiazepines in Table 9.2 on the next page. Instead of prescribing benzodiazepines for chronic fear and anxiety with or without panic episodes, I have found that buspirone (Buspar) helps 80% of people who take it and it is neither numbing nor addicting.

The non-benzo "sleeping pills" (Table 9.3) are more acutely toxic and are close to the benzos in addiction. They commonly disrupt sleep and tend to eliminate dreams that are crucial to our waking up refreshed the next day. See also Chapter 15 on Sleep.

Table 9.2. Benzodiazepine half-life & equivalents

Names	Half-life (hours)	Equivalents (approx. oral)
Alprazolam (trade name Xanax, Xanor)	6-12	0.5 mg
Chlordiazepoxide (Librium)	5–30 (36-200)	25
Clonazepam (Klonopin)	18-50	0.5
Clorazepate (Tranxene)	(36–200)	15
Diazepam (Valium)	20–100 (36-200)	10
Lorazepam (Ativan)	10-20	1
Oxazepam (Serax, Serenid, Serepax)	4-15	20
Temazepam (Restoril, Normison)	8-22	20
Triazolam (Halcion)	2	0.5

Table 9.3. Newer sleep drugs half-life & equivalents

Names	Half-life (hours)	Equivalents (approx. oral)
Zolpidem (Ambien, Stilnoct)	2	20
Eszopiclone (Lunesta)	6	3
Zaleplon (Sonata)	1-2	20
Zopiclone (Zimovane, Imovane)	3-6	15

"MOOD STABILIZERS" AND LITHIUM

"Mood stabilizer" is a marketing term and buzz word for several moderately potent, expensive and toxic anti-epilepsy drugs that are sedating—often to a dysfunctional degree. [29,109,110] That is their only effect on mood. Research and clinical psychiatrist Joanna Moncrieff wrote, "...Contrary to the implication of the term 'mood stabilizer,' there is no evidence that any of these drugs, or any other drugs... help to normalize emotional responses or stabilize mood. ...No drugs have been shown to normalize or smooth out moods, and all drugs prescribed as mood stabilizers are sedative drugs of one form or another." [109] Years ago Big Pharma first got 3 of these anti-epilepsy drugs FDA-approved for treating manic depressive disorder, which classically effects about one person for every 100,000 people—a rare condition indeed. But the large increase in numbers of people taking *most any* psychiatric drug long-term and then *missing doses* or *suddenly stopping* them usually causes withdrawal reactions and syndromes that can mimic such a "roller coaster" emotional experience that are

106

erroneously labeled manic depression, also called "bipolar disorder," and which today is its most likely cause. [25,109,162]

This drug-induced psychiatric drug withdrawal phenomenon mimicking bipolar symptoms and signs may in part explain how it has appeared to be increased above this original 1/100,000 incidence in the general population. Thus the National Institute of Mental Health (NIMH) today estimates that 1 in 83 people at any given time (prevalence) has manic depressive disorder, which is *over* 1200 *times* the original findings of 1/100,000 for it. Even before withdrawal, just taking a mood stabilizer may actually *cause* mood swings—found often with the mood stabilizers gabapentin (Neurontin), topiramate (Topamax), and lamotrigine (Lamictal) . [109] Add one or more other psych drugs, then miss their doses or stop them and it becomes easier to explain how this seeming "bipolar" epidemic is actually a drug-induced artifact usually missed by clinicians and researchers worldwide. [162]

Add another artifact: as mentioned in the other chapters, most clinicians do not screen for PTSD and complex PTSD in their patients and clients, which can mimic other psychiatric disorders, including the commonly misdiagnosed "bipolar." By so misdiagnosing, many to most such people are then mistreated with various psychiatric drugs, including "mood stabilizers" and lithium.

To market their drugs further, drug makers and their paid academic psychiatrists (many of whom own stock in the drug companies that make these drugs) have made up other dimensions on the bipolar theme—"bipolar II" (bipolar I is conventional manic depressive disorder) to mean a kind of manic depression "light," and other vague and unscientific terms as "bipolar spectrum disorders." This drug sales device is a base for their now estimating that 5% of the population fits into such a bipolar spectrum disorder. Bipolar II is said to be manifested by hypo-mania (a non-specific and non-diagnostic term which includes over-optimism, increased energy, pressured speech and activity, and a decreased need for sleep) alternating with periods of "depression." As for bipolar I, with the increased use of toxic psychiatric drugs in these people—from stimulants to antipsychotics—bipolar II is *most often* actually *drug-induced* by clinicians, their patients and others misdiagnosing it. [25,162]

I summarize the toxicity of these common anti-epileptic drugs in Table A.5 in the Appendix on page 206. They commonly cause weight gain, sedation (drowsiness, low energy and fatigue), dizziness, ataxia, upset stomach, serious organ damage, memory loss, headache, difficulty focusing and more. Yet physicians and their assistants continue to prescribe them and other clinicians and some counselors continue to recommend and support their clients taking them. While already of concern in adults, it is of even more concern that millions of children and adolescents are also being so misdiagnosed as "bipolar" and mistreated with these toxic drugs. Unfortunately drug makers have also marketed these drugs for numerous other problems than epilepsy. However, I have found these drugs to be somewhat easier and less emotionally painful to taper and stop than most of the other psychiatric drugs.

In summary, Moncrieff concludes: "... There is no evidence to support the use of a so-called mood stabilizer. ... These drugs suppress mental and physical activities and probably reduce people's emotional responses to their environment in a similar way as neuroleptics [antispychotics]. ... The drugs produce a global state of mental suppression. It seems unlikely that many people would feel that pharmacological restriction of this sort was useful or desirable in the long term."

By contrast, if an antiepileptic drug is needed, I have found that the antiepileptic drug phenytoin (Dilantin) is just as effective for trauma survivors, safer and far less expensive. There is preliminary evidence that taking it for six months to a year may be associated with a correction of the shrinkage of the small but important organ called the hippocampus in the brain found among trauma survivors. [29,30,107] The dose I prescribe is 100 mg by mouth three times daily, and I have seen no associated weight gain or other toxic effects among my patients.

LITHIUM

Also often erroneously called a mood stabilizer, lithium is even more toxic than the others and for this and other reasons it should be eliminated from all use in medicine and psychiatry. [109] It is highly toxic to the brain, nervous system, gastro-intestinal tract, kidneys, and other organs, and often causes weight gain. [10, 25] It is so toxic that its makers recommend that regular blood lithium levels be monitored frequently and long term, which is also expensive. [83] When I see a patient taking lithium and other psych drugs together, it is the first drug that I recommend that they taper and stop taking. When they stop taking it, they often experience eventual improved sleep, mental and physical functioning, and quality of life for most who can handle the emotional pain of and be patient in a full recovery program. Close follow-up monitoring and therapy is crucial.

OPIATES

People use opiates for at least three reasons: pain (physical and/or emotional), recreationally (as a kind of "party" drug), and sometimes as an anti-depressant. For many users opiates give them temporary energy, motivation, and courage—all of which alcohol, other legal and illegal drugs also may provide to a degree.

Some do so for two or more of these reasons. What percentage of short-term opiate users become chemical dependent on them is unknown, although there are an estimated 1.5 million people dependent on them in the USA. When treated for acute pain most patients appear to stop using them when their pain lessens or goes away. [83, 130] Some experience an unpleasant reaction to taking opiates, including nausea, vomiting, and other negative effects (as shown in Table A.6 on page 208 in the Appendix).

Opiate users can find their drugs from various sources, including physicians, friends, relatives, the "street" (drug sellers or "pushers"), and other people's medicine cabinets. Some buy their opiates from enterprising people who first get their opiates from their physicians, usually for physical pain, and then sell them at an inflated price. Opiate dependence can be treated successfully in a number of ways, from Twelve Step fellowships such as Narcotics Anonymous to buprenorphine (Suboxone/Subutex) maintenance. [130]

BUSPIRONE

In my experience buspirone is the least toxic and safest of all the psychiatric drugs. When it first became available I was not impressed. But now with 25 years of clinical experience it has shown that for at least 80% of people it has significant anti-fear and anti-anxiety effects, and it is also an antidepressant [55,99,109,131]. For *chronic* fear and anxiety it is superior to benzodiazapines and barbiturates because it is not mind and emotions numbing or addicting and it has essentially no withdrawal symptoms.

It is now (2011) generic, costing about $4 to $10 for a month's supply in pharmacies with generic drug programs. Similar to antidepressants, it takes up to six weeks of daily use to take a full anti-fear and -anxiety effect, and the dose may need to be increased if the fear and anxiety are not sufficiently reduced by low or standard doses after four to six weeks. After exercise, meditation and right nutrition, it is my drug of choice for many.

A HEALTHIER DRUG FREE LIFE

Not taking psychiatric drugs leaves us free to feel our feelings and be more mentally alert, aware and clear thinking. Being in this natural state we can thereby use these qualities to help us function better in our relationships, on the job, in school, recreation and relaxation – and, if we choose, in our recovery — as we heal from the painful effects of our traumas.

One way to estimate our level of life function is by using the GAF (Global Assessment of Functioning scale from the American Psychiatric Association's *Diagnostic and Statistical Manual*, or *DSM*) as shown in the 4th column in Table 9.1 on page 98 above. The most successfully functioning GAF range is usually from 70 to 100. Only a small percentage of people function from 90 to 100, and most function from 70 and above. Mental health clinicians and physicians use the GAF to objectively and subjectively rate the social, occupational, and psychological functioning of adults, e.g., how well we are handling our various problems-in-living. Look it up online for details.

Most clinicians don't know of the highly significant relationship between psychiatric drug use and having a history of repeated childhood trauma—also called adverse childhood experiences (ACEs). We and others [6,57,173,174] have shown a strong relationship between having a history of ACEs and being prescribed and taking psychiatric drugs. We also found a strong relationship between alcoholism, other chemical dependence and having a significant history of ACEs. [56, 57] For these and other medical populations, finding psychiatric drug use in a patient may lead to further history taking for ACEs and referral to a clinician for evaluation

111

and treatment for the effects of ACEs, including PTSD. The strong graded relationship between mental illness, psychiatric drug use and ACEs that was found in this large sample of the general population supports such an approach to diagnosing and treating many of these patients, as shown on pages 9, 22 and 170.

It is normal to experience stresses and conflicts in life. Add this to having been born into an abusive and or neglectful family and world, and the stress increases to **distress**. And child neglect can increase to physical and emotional abandonment, both of which are kinds of childhood traumas.

Working through these stresses, conflicts and traumas is normal. Whenever we make a mistake we can learn from it and thereby derive and eventually achieve wisdom. In this regard we can remember a basic message of the Serenity Prayer:

> *GOD, GRANT ME THE SERENITY*
> *TO ACCEPT THE THINGS I CANNOT CHANGE;*
> *COURAGE TO CHANGE THE THINGS I CAN;*
> *AND WISDOM TO KNOW THE DIFFERENCE*

Recognizing and finally accepting what we cannot change, we see that it is our false self (ego) that—while it can be a useful assistant to our real self (Child Within)—is our only enemy according to the modern spiritual text *A Course in Miracles* (ACIM). [177,178] Thus there are three blocks to living a fulfilling life:

1) The hurtful effects of the original trauma, which commonly results in various guises of "mental illness,"

2) The resulting misdiagnosis and mistreatment with toxic drugs which thereby shame and disable our real self's functioning, and

3) The above two dynamics leaving the running of our life to the false self, which is unable to do so successfully.

I have addressed these principles of trauma and recovery in several of my books, including especially

• *Healing the Child Within* (Can call it trauma and recovery 101)
• *A Gift to Myself* (the easy-to-read workbook for HtCW)
• *Boundaries and Relationships* (making life safer for self and others)
• *Memory and Abuse* (remembering and healing trauma effects)
• *My Recovery* (an organized and personal plan for healing)
• *The Truth about Depression* (how trauma causes most of it)
• *The Truth about Mental Illness* (how trauma causes most of it)
and in my recent book
• **Wisdom to Know the Difference**: **Core issues in Relationships, Recovery and Living.**

Some have called this current book you hold in your hands an advanced course in healing and recovery—combined with the truth about psychiatric drugs—when compared to my prior books. In each of these I describe what else I have learned from my clinical experience of continuing to assist my patients as they recover and what I have learned from my ongoing interactions with my colleagues and my reading and research. In part I am re-visioning and reframing much of psychiatry and some of psychology in a more clear and reader friendly way.

In the next chapter I address one of the most hurtful practices people can inflict upon one another: forcing them to take toxic psychiatric drugs.

10 Forced Drugging

F orcing people to take psychiatric drugs or to have electro convulsive shock treatment (ECT) is an unfortunate effect of the interplay between our legal, psychiatric and family systems. It is usually a short cut to resolving emotional and behavior problems and it ends up traumatizing those who it tries to help. [179]

Forced drugging occurs along a spectrum from overt (as in court-ordered drugging) to covert (the most common form, e.g., in schools, inside families and in physicians' and some therapists' offices, as well as in hospitals and nursing homes).

FORCED DRUGGING AMONG SPECIAL POPULATIONS

Forced drugging is most often seen among at least 5 groups of people (see Table 10.2 on page 116). The first and most egregious of these involves forcing toxic psychiatric drugs on our children. While forcing drugs on adults is bad enough, doing so on innocent children, whose bodies, brains and nervous systems are in the active and delicate process of development, is approaching, if not outright, being a modern and usually hidden form of child abuse and neglect (e.g., see the work of Peter Breggin and Vera Sherav).

1. CHILDREN AND ADOLESCENTS IN GENERAL

The first category includes children and adolescents in general. Unable to assess, evaluate and address a child's emotional and behavioral pain, parents, school staff and many clinicians mislabel and then help drug their child with toxic psychoactive chemicals. Many of these children will have a trauma history. Among the most often forced are those in foster care, although most of the many millions of these children are outside the foster system.

114

Foster Care Children: Nationwide there are well over 500,000 children in foster care at one time. *More than half* of them have been labeled with "mental illness" or have serious behavior problems. [39, 40] Child welfare authorities routinely resort to drugs to subdue foster children and pacify parents without fully considering non-drug options, and teachers, nurses, doctors and the foster parents *enable* this hurtful process. [141, 142]

Nearly all children before they arrive in foster care have been repeatedly traumatized and in many trauma continues, and most of them likely have PTSD. Already traumatized, rejected and abandoned, the child is mislabeled with having a non-PTSD mental disorder and thereby further traumatized and stigmatized by the clinical and foster care system. Nearly all are given at least one and often several potent and toxic psychiatric drugs. Indeed, studies have shown that children in the foster care system are given these drugs by a factor of 3 to 4 times more often than those who are not in foster care. [141,142,191]

Other Traumatized Children: Unable to care for and handle a difficult yet traumatized child, parents, schools and clinicians similarly mislabel and help drug their children. The child is commonly blamed as being the "problem." These are the majority of children forced to take drugs, and though it is a major problem for them, overall fosters are in the minority.

A Large and Dangerous Problem: In the USA judges can "legally" order controversial drugs to be given to a child over the opposition of the parents. Parents thus allow their children to be drugged for fear of having them taken away by Child Protective Services. In the UK Parents of children diagnosed with ADHD will face jail under proposals in their new Mental Health Bill if they refuse to drug their children. Children do not ask to be drugged. Perhaps not knowing the degree of their toxicity, parents,

Table 10.2 Forced Drugging of Special Populations

Population	Description	Solution
Children & **Adolescents**	Unable to handle a difficult (& often traumatized) child, parents & schools mislabel & help drug their child with toxic chemicals. 4-15X increase in Rx'ing antipsychotics in NJ (Table 10.3 below). "Child = problem" [173,174]	• Stop mislabeling & drugging our kids • Responsibly discipline kids (eg J Lehman program) • Repeal "Teen Screen" program •Ignore drug industry ads & promos
Foster care **Kids** [141,142,191]	Already traumatized, child is further mislabeled & traumatized by clinical & foster system by toxic labels & drugs 3-4x v non-fosters	
Nursing **home**	To sedate (or sometimes stimulate), often end up more sedated & toxic from drugs & other staff mistreatment	Monitor & penalize these abuses
Addiction **treatment**	Staff attempts to help stop some drugs by prescribing other legal psychoactive drugs that are also toxic and addicting [179]	Return to mostly drug free programs, with some exceptions
Court/state **ordered**	A court or a state orders a psychiatric drug under penalty of jail /prison if do not take	• Stop forced drugging • Get clinical/legal advocates support
Prison **inmates**	Some are forced, others seek out legal psychoactive drugs from prison doctors	Open for creative ideas
Drug Stress **Trauma** **Syndrome** [179]	After taking 1 (or usually more) psychiatric drugs, end up feeling more distressed & with a worse quality of life than felt before started the drugs *...a major trauma itself*	• Gradually (months) decrease dose & eventually stop the drug • Psychotherapy for traumas

teachers, clinicians and other authority figures approve, enable and give these toxic drugs to their children.

While we lack exact numbers, we can make some estimates. For example, there may be from **4** to **6 million** children today who have been diagnosed with having "ADHD." Nearly all will likely have been recommended for drug treatment or have been prescribed and given potent stimulant drugs. (Remember that these drugs' effects of stimulation, hyper-stimulation, heart and nervous system damage, growth retardation, and drug addiction now and later in life, are about the same as the effects of illegal methamphetamine made in bathtubs. The only difference is that *illegal* methamphetamine contains additional toxic chemicals.)

We can also estimate that there are from **7 to 10 million** *additional* children and adolescents who have been diagnosed with having various forms of other "mental illness," from "depression" to "bipolar disorder" to "psychosis." Most of these kids and many with "ADHD" grow up in dysfunctional and traumatic families, but most parents and clinicians and school staff don't have the knowledge or skills to recognize and treat their stress-related disorders, such as PTSD. They know only how to focus on the assumed "mental illness". Thus misdiagnosed, most of these children will be mistreated with potent and toxic psychiatric drugs. Many of these drugs have not been approved by the FDA for kids and teens. Some, such as antidepressants, have been *disapproved* by the FDA and its equivalent in other countries, due to their high tendency to *cause* suicidality and other violent behavior (see Appendix A.1-2 on pages 199-202). But parents, clinicians, school staff, courts and other authority figures, acting as kinds of legal drug pushers, continue to force millions of our children to take them daily with no consequences to their negligence and pharmacological abuse. [25,142,179,191]

ANTIPSYCHOTICS FORCED ON CHILDREN

The most toxic, dangerous and mind numbing drugs are the antipsychotics. As an example, investigative journalist Ed Silverman has investigated and exposed how over the 8-year period from 2000 to 2007 antipsychotic drugs have been given in rapidly-increasing numbers to children (see Table 10.3). And these numbers, in per-thousand dollar amounts, are for **New Jersey Medicaid**-paid and -treated **children** *only*. Note that this is for only *one* state (New Jersey) and *one* funding source (Medicaid) for a total taxpayer cost of 73 million dollars. [191]

Table 10.3 Antipsychotics given to Children paid by NJ Medicaid (*only*) from Ed Silverman. All $ numbers are in **$1,000s** [191]

Drug	2000	2001	2002	2003	2004	2005	2006	2007
Abilify	$ 0	$ 0	$ 0	$ 309**	$ 1,420	$ 3,081	$ 4,984	$ 6,115
Geodon	$ 0	$ 41.5	$ 129	$ 212	$ 295	$ 390	$ 437	$ 397
Zyprexa	$ 751	$ 1,270	$ 1,504	$ 1,719	$ 1,594	$ 1,282	$ 1,271	$ 1,107
Risperdal	$1,954	$3,259	$4,022	$ 4,885	$ 4,986	$ 5,419	$ 5,797	$ 5,522
Seroquel	$ 150	$ 422	$ 905	$ 1,556	$1,882	$2,375	$2,732	$3,011
Thorazine	$ 36	$ 41	$ 36	$ 26	$ 14	$ 14	$ 15	$ 18
Haldol	$ 6.6	$ 8.6	$ 13	$ 18	$ 17	$ 13.7	$ 8	$ 9.5

No one may know for sure, but the number is big. By "big" we're *not* talking about hundreds or even thousands of our children. It is highly likely that **multi-millions** of U.S. children are being force-fed these neuro- and metabolic-toxic chemicals (Fig 14.1, p 182).

Silverman's expose' represents only the tip of the iceberg. It reports *only antipsychotics* and *does **not*** include:

1) Children given stimulants such as Ritalin, 2) Those given antidepressants, 3) Those given benzodiazepines, 4) Those given "mood stabilizers" (which are actually potent anti-convulsants.) It also does **not** include **non-Medicaid**-covered children in New Jersey **or** any of the other 49 states in the USA.

If there are 4 to 6 million kids with "ADHD" and another 7 to 10 million with other "mental disorders," there may be from 11 (4 plus 7) to 16 (6 plus 10) million, most of whom have been misdiagnosed as being "mentally ill" and mistreated with toxic drugs. This amounts to from **13 to 19%** of all of our children. This information is waving a big red flag in front of us. From what we know about the effects of trauma on child development, we are headed for potentially big trouble by so re-traumatizing these large numbers of our children. [162, 179]

TEENSCREEN:
BIG PHARMA & BIG GOVERNMENT INVADE THE CLASSROOM

As another guise of forced drugging our children, one of the most insidious and dangerous is the TeenScreen program. Its admirable-on-the-surface goal is to identify "mental illness," especially "depression" and "bipolar disorder" among our children and teens, and then to "treat" it. But it has numerous potential flaws, methodological errors, and big red flags. It is funded and promoted by: 1) Big Pharma and 2) Big government, and promoted by 3) the New Freedom Commission funded by the former two Bigs and composed of members paid under the table by Big Pharma, including 4) Seemingly independent mental health advocacy groups such as the National Alliance for the Mentally Ill, the American Psychiatric Association, and Columbia University School of Medicine's Psychiatry Department—all three of these are also substantially funded by the former two Bigs. All of these connections loudly broadcast a *conflict of interest.*

There is no scientific proof that TeenScreen will work or has ever worked. Teen Screen's hidden agendas are 1) To get more people (now as children, soon to be adults) diagnosed with mental illness and onto Big Pharma's psych drugs long-term or for life, and 2) To "dumb them down," to give Big Government more power, with more people thereby dependent on both Bigs [141,142].

More problems: TeenScreen is the result of heavy lobbying allowed by our federal congress for our tax money. Its screening interviewers are *untrained* lay people, *not* licensed clinicians with expertise in recognizing and treating mental, emotional and behavioral problems. It has an 84% *false positive* rate, which means that out of every 100 children and teens who are identified by TeenScreen as "being suicidal," 84 are in fact normal.

The ultimate tragedy of TeenScreen is that increasing numbers of our children will be misdiagnosed and mis-labeled. That error alone would be damaging enough. But then they will likely be mistreated with antidepressants and given other toxic psych drugs. Warning labels have already been out for years in the USA, the UK and throughout Europe that antidepressant drugs *increase* the incidence of suicidality among children and teens by a factor 2 to 3 times that found for those given placebo controls. But many to most clinicians do not acknowledge and use that obvious and crucial information in their decision making about this toxic effect of antidepressants. These drugs also increase the incidence of homicide. Closely connected to TeenScreen is the **Texas Medication Algorithm Project** (TMAP), which is an older version of TeenScreen that has been used for years on adults, and also financed by Big Pharma (this time by Lilly, Pfizer, and J&J).

I summarize the TeenScreen components and dynamics in Table 10.4. With no evidence of a lasting benefit for children, and every reason to be suspicious of a subjective, rigged questionnaire designed to stir self-doubt among impressionable children—this appears to be a mental-illness-encouragement and **expansion** program to sell and hook children and future adults on their drugs.

Table 10.4 TeenScreen : the Bigs invade High School

Area/Action	People & Methods	Problems/Conflicts of interest
Origin	David Shaffer MD Columbia U **DISC** [19] development group, & **numerous others**	Consultant to at least Roche, GSK, & Wyeth
Made into	1) TeenScreen 14/22 questions, screens for "depression," "bipolar," A&D 2) BSADepr 8/22 questions	Untrained interviewers made 84% false positives;[20] e.g., 27% are "suicidal" 16% predictability
Funded & promoted by...	Big Pharma, Big Gov, NFC [21], & paid MH Orgs [22], APA, Columbia U	Major & numerous, incl. controversial TMAP [23]
Overt goal	Identify "mental illness" & "treat" it	Numerous. No scientific proof will work. See below
Hidden agenda	Get more people, now children (soon adults), on our drugs long-term to lifelong. "Dumb them down" to give big Gov, etc more power	Heavy lobbying of congress for $ for TeenScreen, BSAD, & SMHinc
Resulting Problems	Screened → "Diagnosed" → Referred Psychiatrist/MD/NP prescribes psychiatric drugs long term	Mislabeling, misRxing ADPs→ 2-3x suicidality, DSTS possible, see Chap X

---

[19] DISC = Diagnostic Interview Schedule for Children, 22 questions for depression.
[20] Of every 100 referred to a clinician as "suicidal," 84 are in fact normal.
[21] NFC = New Freedom Comission (chaired by MF Hogan, NY MH director, consultant for Janssen pharma & has promoted TMAP, with its big Pharma & Gov connections; conflicts-of-interest abound).
[22] NAMI, NMHAssoc, NAsMHPlan&AdvCouncil, FedFamsforChildren'sMH, NCouncil for ComBehavHC, NMHAssoc, BazelonCtrforMHLaw, most funded by big Pharma & Gov big "donations" = $ales & profits
[23] TMAP = Texas Medication Algorithm Project ↔ Lilly, Pfizer, J&J, screening program & flow chart to promote & Rx psych drugs= bigger $ales & profits

Of course, the real winner are the Bigs, especially Pharma, who are the covert sponsors of this subversive mental screening.

Some Ways Out of this dilemma include:
• Stop mislabeling and drugging our kids; instead give them our healthy attention, evaluation and boundaries as needed.
• When appropriate, responsibly discipline them with healthy boundaries and limits; for especially troublesome children, clinician James Lehman has an effective approach [96].
• Repeal the "teen screen" law if it becomes one.
• Ignore drug industry advertisements and promotions.
• Stop using television and video games as babysitters.

2. NURSING HOME PATIENTS

A large percentage of people in extended care and nursing homes are also being drugged. These are not usually simple sleeping aids or ordinary medicines. They are commonly any and all of the chemical cocktails which often include one or more antidepressants, antipsychotics, benzodiazepines, anticonvulsants ("mood stabilizers") and now toxic anti-dementia drugs.

To control their patients' expression of emotion and other behaviors some of the nursing home staff use these drugs without clear informed consent on these vulnerable people to sedate, subdue, or chemically restrain them. By their toxicity, this kind of forced drugging often over-sedates, *or* over-stimulates or agitates them, which promotes giving them more sedating benzodiazepines.

A way out of this form of chemical abuse and trauma could be to monitor these facilities and penalize those who violate safe and humane practices.

3. ADDICTION AND DRUG TREATMENT FACILITIES

Common sense was in place in most addiction and drug treatment facilities over the 50-year span from about 1940 through 1990, founded within the wisdom of Alcoholics Anonymous. Unfortunately, from 1990 through today toxic and addictive drugs are routinely and freely given by in- and out-patient addiction treatment facilities to people with chemical dependence (drug and alcohol addiction). There are few places where this strange and counter-intuitive practice is not carried on today (e.g., Willingway Hospital in Statesboro, Ga). These treatment programs usually give little attention to screening their patients for PTSD. In my decades of assisting countless alcoholics and other chemical dependent people, I have yet to find one of them who grew up in a healthy or non-abusive family. The research evidence bears out my observations: 153 studies by independent authors worldwide on 261,596 chemical dependents, childhood trauma survivors, and their controls that shows a highly significant relationship between chemical dependence and repeated childhood and later trauma (see Table 1.2 on page 10 and Table 6.2 on page 60).

Since 1990 I have seen increasing numbers of patients with alcoholism and other drug dependence who have been prescribed one and usually multiple psychoactive drugs, most of which do not help them significantly in their recoveries. These toxic drugs have made many of them worse, and I have seen a number of them to have the painful Drug Stress Trauma Syndrome (DSTS, described in Chapter 7 on page 67). A **way out** of this kind of forced drugging is to return to providing mostly drug-free alcohol and drug treatment programs, with few exceptions for selected patients.

4. COURT AND STATE ORDERS

Under the threat of jail or prison, a court judge or state authority figure orders the person to take whatever drug(s) a psychiatrist prescribes. The purpose or reason for doing so is usually that the person has 1) committed a crime for which a drug may be given to help control their behavior, or 2) is a danger to themselves or others and they are usually diagnosed as having a serious mental illness, such as a psychosis or are suicidal or are a homicidal threat.

When someone is a danger to themselves or others, but have not committed a crime for which they can be arrested and held, families and societies look for and try to sort out the best alternatives to handle the problem. A problem is that in most cases all the treatment alternatives are not seriously taken into consideration. In some situations, giving a drug as a kind of "chemical straightjacket" to a violent person may be appropriate. But too often a *non-violent* person is taken or sent to a hospital psychiatric unit or to a psychiatrist, where they will often be given psychiatric drugs *against their will* or *without* clear *informed consent.* [80,81] Nearly all such patients are given a mental disorder diagnosis without taking an adequate childhood and later trauma history and doing a careful screening for PTSD. The automatic next step is giving potent injected or oral psychiatric drugs without giving patients clear warning about the likelihood of toxic effects (usually called "side effects," which tries to hide the truth about their toxicity), including the high likelihood of a bothersome-to-severe drug withdrawal syndrome should they miss a dose or more or try to stop taking the drug(s). [111]

Psychiatric Advanced Directive: In most states of the USA there is available a mechanism that *may* help prevent people from being forcibly drugged or given ECT. [65] It is called a **psychiatric advanced**

directive, wherein the person fills out a several-page form by stating their wishes and the form is signed by a clinician, certifying that the person is not in a psychotic state when they signed the document. Whether future psychiatrists will honor it is dependent on their clinical knowledge, integrity and compassion. It may also be helpful for the concerned person to remember Joseph Campbell's classic statement that I mentioned earlier, *"The difference between a psychotic and a mystic is that the mystic knows who not to talk to."*

5. PRISON INMATES

Prison inmates are about the only population where many of them seek out and ask for antipsychotics and antidepressants. This may be because around 80% of prison inmates are alcoholics and/or other chemical dependent, and essentially all are survivors of repeated childhood and later trauma, and 50% or more are sociopaths. There is something about this group and the unsafe and unhealthy prison environment that contributes to the fact that these inmates voluntarily seek out and take potent and toxic psych drugs such as antipsychotics and antidepressants—drugs that the general population does not generally pursue and which therefore usually have no value on the street black market.

Even so, a percentage of prison inmates are forced to take antipsychotics to act as chemical straitjackets to help control belligerent or dangerous behavior and/or to prevent withdrawal. While it may be hard to have sympathy for many among this population, they do add another dimension to the spectrum of people who are forced to take psych drugs

Given the above, it becomes clearer that the phenomenon and practice of forced drugging is far more common and prevalent than we thought. It occurs across a spectrum from overt to covert, as shown in Figure 10.4 below. The overt kind is the more obvious.

And those included under the covert category given the above descriptions, may now be more visible and understandable to us.

Table 10.4 Forced Drugging Spectrum Dynamics

Overt	Covert	Drug- & System-Induced
Court ordered	Parents, schools, and clinicians to children	Political (power) and clinical drug-induced
Nearly all **psychiatric units** and **clinics** overtly push or require psych drugs in all patients	Traumatized and foster care children	Viscous cycle of habituation/addiction, as in the phenomena of spellbinding (page 210) & withdrawal
Referring to next—> 2 cells: Both under covert spectrum commonly force drugs on patients that is overt in these settings	**Nursing home** patients	DSTS occurs in many [179]
	Health insurance enforced (including Medicare & Medicaid)	Psych clinics and units

We can introduce a third kind of forced drugging, even more covert, wherein the *force* comes from the *drug itself* through its *spellbinding* and other toxic effects and from the clinical and political system that delivers or pushes the drug onto and into the vulnerable and unknowing person. Inherent in this combination of the drug(s) and the system is a subtle yet frequently toxic interaction that can ultimately be an actual traumatic experience for the patient, who ends up feeling worse and with a worse quality of life, than when they started taking the psychiatric drug. I call this condition the *Drug Stress Trauma Syndrome*, which I addressed in the Chapter 7. Having read this chapter, I now ask if BigPharma and their many enablers are *pushing* their *legal* drugs?

11   Legal Drug Pushing?
THE ORIGIN AND DISTRIBUTION OF PSYCHIATRIC DRUGS

"This is all marketing dressed up to look like science"
John Abramson MD et al from documentary, *Money Talks* [1,2]

As a person labeled with a "mental illness" or as a clinician who assists people with their associated pain, or as a friend or relative, it may be useful to know what lies behind, around and underneath the industry and groups that drive the misdiagnosis and mistreatment.

The legal drug industry is a business. Their main reason for finding, making and selling their drugs is to *make money for* their employees and investors. They deserve to make a profit, but to sell their wares they use all kinds of methods—from legal and even illegal to unethical. [8,9] These methods—also called marketing devices—are many which I outline in Table 11.1 and discuss below.

To sell their drugs they have to make them appear as if they are more effective to combat illness than they are toxic to the body and mind. [1, 2, 8, 9] Ideally, their advantages will outweigh their disadvantages, commonly described as a risk/benefit ratio. The lower the *toxicity* or *risk* of a given drug may be—when compared to its *advantage* or *benefit*—the safer and better usually is the drug. The main problem with psychiatric drugs is that they have a serious and detrimental *high risk/benefit ratio,* [10,187] as I describe in this book and in *The Truth about Depression* and *The Truth about Mental Illness.*

A COMPLEX WEB OF INFLUENCE AND CONTROL
In part because psychiatric drugs are so ineffective and toxic, their makers have infiltrated several areas of our lives that were *previously* independent and respected. [25] These areas include the

Table 11.1 Common Psychiatric Drug Marketing Devices

Marketing Device	Description	Message
Buzz words - e.g., **"Evidence based,"** **"Science"** -terms often misused	These are buzz words or sound bytes; often made up and misused by Big Pharma & the other Bigs (Government, Insurance, Academia, Professional Groups)	May be used positively (patient care, improved health) or negatively (marketing, influence, power, manipulation)
DSM * (diagnostic "bible" or manual of the APA – American Psychiatric Assn) infiltrated by several, including BigPharma	Based on symptoms and surface experiences, not on problems or causes. Contaminated by its authors' being paid by Big Pharma, who often influences them to make up new "diseases" or "disorders"	Descriptions of disorders are determined mostly by APA committee *consensus voting*, & less on basic or clinical science.
Drug's **generic** & **trade names**	Both are made up to sell the drug. Another marketing device.	No science behind the names.
Medical/psychiatry **journals** **	Over half of authors have conflicts of interest, esp. those who receive drug money or stocks. Most journals are largely subsidized by drug ads.	We can't trust most medical journals to tell us the truth, including NEJM & JAMA
Published clinical **drug trials** *	Most (at least 80%) report positive results only. Most negative trial results are never published. Conclusions are often erroneous or distorted.	90% of drug trials and studies are funded by the drug companies marketing the specific drug. Most data are hidden from the public and often from the authors who write about the drugs.
Drug ads in news-letters, magazines & journals	Pharma fills psychiatric & medical journals with ads similar to what we see in magazines & newspapers, including enticements & deceptions	We can't trust media ads to tell us the truth. No one watches out for consumers

Marketing Device	Description	Message
Organizations ProfessionalGroups	Many are in bed with and subsidized by Big Pharma and the other Bigs.	Example groups: NAMI, APA, congressional lobbies.
Political lobbyists	Opinion leaders & lawmakers lobbied include politicians, authorities, physicians, NIH, CDC, FDA, NIMH, and their neuroscience researchers and staff.	*2 lobbyists* exist for every 1 politician, which is greater than for banking, oil, or any other industry. Federal trade secret laws allow drug companies to hide the negatives about drugs
TV Drug commercials	One of a long list of inappropriate laws enacted by congress, whose members are usually paid for votes through lobbies by Big Pharma.	Insidious influences, empty claims, false hope, minimize toxic drug effects
Drug "Reps" (attractive, perky "cheerleader" sales people, most with no formal or background drug or science training)	There are 90,000 drug sales reps in the USA, or 1 per 4 physicians. Thousands of drugs are available, & physicians can't remember the names or details of all. Rep promotes their co's drugs, leaves samples to hook MD & patient.	Doctors can't trust the information they transmit verbally or in writing to them. Yet many rely on this misinformation for how they practice medicine & psychiatry.
Psychiatric drug samples left by drug reps	A major marketing tool to get physicians and patients hooked on their drug.	Over half are paid for by Big Pharma's drug promotional money (outside their "charity" budget).
Inherent psychiatric **drug withdrawal**	Nearly all drugs have a bothersome to severe withdrawal. Kept secret from physicians, patients & the public by Big Pharma & its drug reps	Usually misinterpreted as "relapse" or "another disorder" for which more drugs or ECT are prescribed

"**Continuing** *** **Medical Education**" CME	70% by BigPharma Free seminars & dinners, etc. Nearly all promote drug use as only or best treatment.	Can't trust these sessions for accurate medical information
Medical school researchers, faculty and authors*	University and medical school based authors are commonly paid by Big Pharma.	Their publications are usually marketing dressed up to look like science.
"**Expert opinion**" speaches & writing "KOL" = Key Opinion Leader	At least 60% of experts who write diagnostic and treatment guidelines are paid by Big Pharma. $20 billion are spent on marketing drugs, which is *twice* the money spent on research.	Can't trust these for accurate medical information. These publications are usually more marketing dressed up to look like science.
Websites about illness or drugs	At least 80% of websites on drugs or disorders are secretly funded by Big Pharma.	Difficult to find objective ones. See, e.g., ahrp.blogspot.com crbestbuydrugs.com
Physicians & other **clinicians** prescribing & recommending	Much of education & practice are influenced by the Bigs, promoting drug over non-drug healing aids. Their unawareness of drug toxicity & ineffectiveness brings major sales.	These become the best drug marketing device in which Big Pharma can invest, which they do: $30,000 PER year PER doctor
Psychiatry units in hospitals	Do a cursory, usually incomplete evaluation (no trauma history), followed by (mis)diagnosis & (mis)treatment with toxic drugs ± ECT; part of the viscious cycle	Discharge patient on toxic & addicting drugs to 10-15 minute sessions with a drug oriented psychiatrist ± longer with a counselor

*DSM is infiltrated by researchers and physicians paid by Big Pharma. **NEJM = New England Journal of Medicine, JAMA = Journal of the American Medical Association. ***CME=continuing medical (or psychiatric) education; commonly has a conflict-of-interest in what it presents as "evidence-based" education programs. KOLs = Key Opinion Leaders; ECT = Electro Convulsive/Shock Therapy integrity and the truth-seeking relationship among scientists, researchers, physicians, medical schools, continuing medical education, professional organizations, clinical trials, and medical journals—to name a few [1,2]. This invasion and extensive infiltration of our health care system is part of a complex web of influence and control on our clinical helping professionals, including the physicians and psychiatrists and their aides who prescribe these drugs—and even psychologists, social workers, and counselors who enable these physicians by supporting or even recommending that their clients take these drugs (see Figure 11.1, p. 133). This is ultimately an insidious web of influence, control and harm on and over our patients and clients—people of all ages and their families.

BIG PHARMA

The primary focal point or hub of this web is Big Pharma, which consists of the several large and highly influential drug companies worldwide. Individually and collectively these drug producers act in legal and sometimes illegal and unethical ways not only to sell their drugs but often to force them onto unsuspecting patients of all ages and their families. [8,9] To accomplish this goal, they interact with numerous others in the web (Figure 11.1), especially the other "Bigs" (Big Government, Big Insurance, Big Academia and Big Professional Groups). Big Pharma's primary method is by paying money to members of these other Bigs directly and indirectly (and sometimes under the table)—usually their physicians, researchers, administrators and politicians. They pay *directly* through lobbying by their "donations" to politicians, and directly and *indirectly* for various "services," "grants," "support" or "subsidies" to scientists, physicians and administrators—as well as groups and institutions. The now paid-off politicians then make laws that are usually in the favor of BigPharma's legal drug pushing, e.g., TV ads for drugs. The other paid-off people then promote and prescribe the drugs.

KEY OPINION LEADERS

An especially effective way for Big Pharma to influence and control our health care system is by paying and controlling "key opinion leaders" who the former editor of *The New England Journal of Medicine* Marcia Angell MD describes as being, "...highly influential [medical school] faculty physicians—referred to by the industry as 'thought-leaders' or 'key opinion leaders' (KOLs). These are the people who write textbooks and medical journal articles, issue practice guidelines (treatment recommendations), sit on FDA and other governmental advisory panels, head professional societies, and speak at the innumerable meetings and dinners that take place every year to "teach" clinicians about prescription drugs." [7, 8] I summarize 3 KOLs in Table 11.2 and contrast them with 3 KOLs from nearly a century ago. Read over Table 11.2, then return here to the text.

KOL Joseph Biederman and his colleagues and followers appear to have set back child and adolescent psychiatry to the dark ages. Instead of using tried-and-true healthy parenting, combined with new discoveries about child development and childhood trauma recovery, Beiderman et al have ignored these and appear to have actually harmed the children and families they purport to treat. [98]

Bruce Levine writes, "In America's assembly-line medicine, drug prescriptions are routinely written without any exploration of commonsense reasons as to why a child might be behaving problematically. • Is the child resentful over a perceived injustice? • Is the child experiencing deep emotional pain? • Is the child simply bored? • Does the child feel powerless? • Does the child have low self-worth because of a lack of life skills and thus behaves immaturely so no expectations are placed on them? • Is the child starving for attention? • Has the child lost respect for his or her parents because these adults have not acted like adults? • Has the child's basic physical needs — such as proper nutrition,

Figure 11.1 The Complex Web of Influence and Control

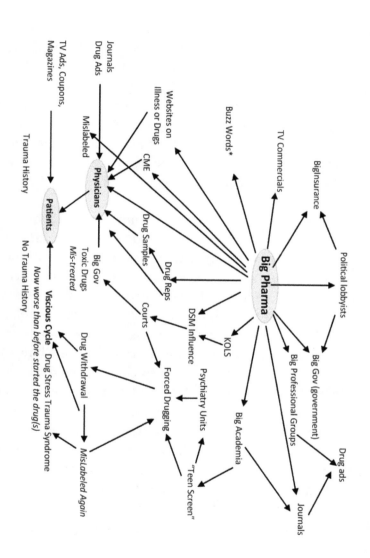

Conflicts-of-interest are *rampant* throughout this web

physical activity, or sleep—not been met? Routinely, few if any of these areas are explored before a prescription is written." [98]

Many troubled and disruptive children—most of whom are being mis-parented, abused or neglected—are sometimes destructive to themselves or others. Any attempt to understand them by consulting most psychiatrists and some other clinicians will likely be corrupted by this financial and/or educational dependence on drug companies, which have a vested interest in promoting all emotional and behavioral difficulties as diseases that can be fixed with drugs. Plus the corruption among school teachers who want to have their children drugged to make their job easier.

On another KOL, Marcia Angell [9] commented, "Emory benefited from [Charles] Nemeroff's grants and other activities, and that raises the question of whether its lax oversight was influenced by its own conflicts of interest. As reported by Gardiner Harris in *The New York Times*, Nemeroff himself had pointed out his value to Emory in a 2000 letter to the dean of the medical school, in which he justified his membership on a dozen corporate advisory boards by saying: "Surely you remember that Smith-Kline Beecham Pharmaceuticals donated an endowed chair to the department and there is some reasonable likelihood that Janssen Pharmaceuticals will do so as well. In addition, Wyeth-Ayerst Pharmaceuticals has funded a Research Career Development Award program in the department, and I have asked both AstraZeneca Pharmaceuticals and Bristol-Myers Squibb to do the same. Part of the rationale for their funding our faculty in such a manner would be my service on these boards." This amounts to at least 5 drug companies that had infiltrated Nemeroff's psychiatry department up until he was exposed. [9,70,127]

In addition to being unethical, psychiatrists such as these violated federal rules designed to prevent and police conflicts of

Table 11.2. Key Opinion Leaders: the tip of the iceberg in psychiatry & medicine

KOL examples	Observations	Money involvement
Joseph Biederman MD Harvard psychiatrist	With no scientific evidence & ignoring normal child development, he promoted children two years old & younger having "bi-polar disorder" & treating them with a toxic drug cocktail, not approved by FDA. He saw nothing unethical about doing this.	Received > $1.6 million over 7 years from Big Pharma
Alan Schatzberg MD Stanford psychiatrist APA President	Tested toxic abortion-inducing drug RU-486 ("mifepristone") from Corcept Therapeutics to treat psychotic depression. He saw nothing unethical about doing this. Stanford removed him as principle investigator. Edited a drug-pushing book with CN below:	He controlled over $6 million in the drug co.
Charles Nemeroff MD Emory Univ. psychiatry; chair now at U Miami	Promoting toxic psychiatric drugs, did not disclose $100,000/year pay from GSK over 5 years, while Emory & NIH limited it to $10,000 /year. One year he reported $9,999 when he received $171,000. Emory removed him as psychiatry chair & banned him NIH grants for 2 years. Yet Emory received one third of his grant money. He saw nothing unethical about doing this.	Received $500,000 over 5 years from 1 drug co. (GSK alone); got $2.8 mil from 12 others)
Summary for 2009 The 3 above KOLs	These 3 may represent the tip of the iceberg among academic psychiatrists, as KOLs are in bed with Big Pharma, promoting toxic drugs that do not work well. They claim that mental illness is caused by genetically inherited disorders of brain chemistry when there is no definitive proof. They ignore other forms of treatment than drugs & ECT.	The above conflicts of interest are usual among academic psychiatrists

interest such as being *paid* by Big Pharma's *drug money while receiving* federal *research funds* that are often *supposed to evaluate* the very *drug made by* the *paying* drug maker. For example, Beiderman was researching the amphetamine kiddie-cocaine drug

Strattera and the anti-psychotic Risperdal *for children* with federal money while allegedly being paid over and under the table by Eli Lilly and Johnson and Johnson, respectively, for supposedly objectively studying their products. [98]

Levine continues, "Mental health treatment in the United States is now a multibillion-dollar industry, and all the rules of industrial complexes apply. Not only does Big Pharma have influential psychiatrists such as Biederman in their pocket, virtually every mental health institution from which doctors, the press, and the general public receive their mental health information is *financially interconnected* with Big Pharma. The American Psychiatric Association, psychiatry's professional organization, is hugely dependent on drug company grants, and this is also true for the National Alliance for the Mentally Ill (NAMI) and other so-called consumer organizations. Harvard and other prestigious university psychiatry departments take millions of dollars from drug companies, and the National Institute of Mental Health funds researchers who are financially connected with drug companies."[98]

These findings show us several examples of the dangers of anyone relying on Key Opinion Leaders to keep us updated on their take on the truth about mental illness and psychiatric drugs. When realized, these dangers significantly harm medicine and psychiatry and their patients and families. They harm them by the enmeshed relationship between Big Pharma and the KOLs who it pays to promote their pseudo-science and sell their drugs. These dangers manifest especially when Big Pharma and its KOLs do any of the following:

1) Make up illnesses and unproven theories about mental, emotional and behavioral experiences in the name of "science" and "evidence" (see Table 11.1 on page 128 above on Buzz Words).

2) Ignore normal child development, unhealthy parenting, and childhood trauma and neglect as being important factors in causing emotional and behavioral distress in people of all ages.

3) Act in inappropriate, unethical or greedy ways to take advantage of their position in teaching and patient care.

4) Enable and even promote Big Pharma to infiltrate and harmfully influence medicine and psychiatry and their patient care delivery.

This is in contrast to the three Key Opinion Leaders (who were not called that) from nearly a century ago (Table 11.3). Among Freud, Jung and Ferenczi, all of whom contributed to psychology and psychiatry, only Freud had a similar conflict of interest to those of today. Given the above and more, the very naming and identification of KOLs as being positive for us folks is suspect. Who so named them as a KOL? If a KOL doesn't validate and promote what Big Pharma wants, they are usually dropped from a Big Pharma paid lecture circuit, which I have observed first hand.

Often a KOL speaker will bring a prepared talk, only to have a BigPharma staff who is present at the talk to censor their slides and illustrations by inserting those pre-made and brought by Big Pharma to the presentation that show only the positives of their product.

DEFINING OPINION

The central term in KOL is "opinion." An opinion is a belief, theory, claim or judgment that is strongly held—but *without* actual *proof* of its truth. It is *not a fact*. Opinions are based on the person or group's current view or understanding of a subject. It may be true, close to the truth or have no basis in the truth. It may be a simple projection based only on the opinion-giver's wants, needs, personal welfare or unconscious unhealed traumas. The *DSM* is another clear example of this principle (pages 12, 17, 83, 179). [185]

Table 11.3. KOLs: 3 examples from the past

KOL examples	Observations	Money involvement
Sigmund Freud MD 1856-1939 neurologist	In 1896 Freud summarized his 18 patients with PTSD, which he called "hysteria," caused by childhood trauma (CSA). After monetary pressure from his peers, he recanted & made up the Oedipus complex that blamed the child. He, Jung and others named and described the unconscious, repetition compulsion, & dream analysis.	Freud's conflict-of-interest : he retracted his trauma facts & *made up* the Oedipal theory.
Carl Jung MD 1675-1961 psychiatrist	Expanded Freud inner circle's work into the transpersonal, including archetypes & the collective unconscious.	
Sandor Ferenczi MD 1873-1933 psychiatrist	Believed his patients' accounts of CSA, having verified them through other patients in the same family and eventually broke from Freud. Made other important contributions, including empathy importance & other trauma recovery concepts.	By contrast, Ferenczi usually believed his patients' trauma history
Summary **1896 present**	**These 3 KOLs are examples of the positive potential of psychiatry and psychology even today**	**Less conflicts of interest**

It is a sad day when scientists and physicians are so influenced, manipulated and even controlled in this way to bypass and even surrender their integrity, to get more money, control and recognition instead of making a real contribution to their patients' health and their own profession.

Next to Big Pharma and its KOLs, Big Orgs (Big Professional Groups) play an influential role in helping Big Pharma market their drugs and misinformation about them. "This ... is the tip of the iceberg on conflict of interest in medicine," said Dr. Daniel Carlat, a psychiatrist at the Tufts University School of Medicine who edits a newsletter about psychiatry and writes a blog about conflicts of interest (see carlatpsychiatry.blogspot.com).

THE ROLE OF BIG GOVERNMENT

Big Government is another key player in pushing psychiatric drugs. Bigger government means less individual freedom in a number of ways. [27] BigGov (including the US Congress, the Food and Drug Administration, the Drug Enforcement Administration and the National Institutes of Health and Mental Health) interacts with and supports the other Bigs, especially through all of their numerous conflicts-of-interest with BigPharma, whose many influences and psychiatric drugs also stifle our individual freedom and creativity by their brain disabling and mind-numbing actions. [25] As but one example, since the advent of government-funded Medicaid in 1965 more and more people, *including abused and neglected children*, and especially indigent or low income trauma survivors with PTSD have been repeatedly misdiagnosed with various "mental illnesses" and mistreated with psychiatric drugs that make them worse. I have seen many such patients who are as dependent and addicted to their state and federal taxpayer-funded welfare *disability entitlements* as they are in a vicious cycle to their numerous drugs—from nicotine to alcohol to psychiatric drugs. Most were in a revolving-door cycle with other clinicians who—like BigGov—enabled their non-self-supporting and unfortunately non-productive life choices and lifestyle. They and many of their enablers did not and may still not know what had happened to them and that small government (which allows us more personal freedom overall) and taking no psychiatric drugs give us all more opportunities and personal power to live, heal and transcend their unhealthy dependence on Big Gov. For them to find a clinician who is not a further enabler of their unhealthy dependence on BigGov in these ways is difficult but possible if they can muster enough motivation, patience and persistence to fully recover. (see p 224)

THE WAY OUT – MAINTAIN FULL AWARENESS

What can we do to surmount the reality of this legal drug pushing on to us as clinicians, patients, and their family members and friends? For sake of space, I summarize it in outline form below and in my books *The Truth About Depression* and *The Truth about Mental Illness*.

Distrust most medical and psychiatry journals *and* popular print media *and* TV regarding what they say about psychiatric drugs. Notice how rampant and indoctrinating their advertisements are trying to sell the drugs and how *rare* these journals address non-drug healing and recovery aids—from psychotherapy and counseling to nutrition, exercise, meditation, yoga, spirituality, prayer and nutritional supplements—to help people recover from the effects of trauma.

Question your physicians and all other clinicians about *any* of your concerns. Do you have to do all of their biddings?

Leave their office or decline their drugs at any one or especially more of these "**red flags**": [1,2]

- they give you samples of psychiatric drugs;
- you see any drug sales representatives in waiting room or office;
- you repeatedly have a long wait (more than 30 minutes);
- you have a short visit (less than 20 minutes);
- they do little or no listening to your concerns or story; and
- they prescribe drugs as their only treatment recommendation.

See Table A.8 on page 215 for more marketing myths and Chapter 14 -page 170 for a summary of the process of healing and recovery.

In the next chapter I address some principles of how, if you consider or choose, to taper and stop taking one or more psychiatric drugs.

12   Stopping Psychiatric Drugs

There are several important and valid reasons to avoid beginning or, once started, to stop taking psychiatric drugs.

1) Nearly all psychiatric drugs produce adverse or toxic effects from over-sedation (most common) or over-stimulation to mind numbing to weight gain and diabetes to inability to have an orgasm (anorgasmia).

2) By doing the above and more, most of these drugs are toxic to the brain and body. I have summarized this principle in the accompanying tables, backed up by numerous references in research and clinical psychiatrist Peter Breggin's 2008 book *Brain-Disabling Treatments in Psychiatry*, others' observations, and in my books. [25,81,109,173,174]

3) Similar to alcohol and other sedative drugs, these drugs tend to numb our feelings and emotions, making it difficult to impossible to use these helpful emotional cues in handling our lives more constructively.

4) Nearly all psych drugs have addictive properties, making it difficult for most people to stop taking them due to their painful withdrawal symptoms.

5) When they do help, they are only lessening symptoms associated with the diagnosed or assumed "mental illness." Psychiatric drugs do not treat or cure any specific illness or disorder. [25,109]

6) Instead, they lessen symptoms by their "shotgun" effects whereby they impact almost all body and neural systems, and not by a single bullet aimed at a single symptom, problem or target, such as penicillin works against specific bacterial infections. This fact helps explain more of their toxicity (see pages 141 and 142).

7) Due to their toxicity, over time they tend to worsen many to most people's original symptoms and problems and not make them better. I call this phenomenon the Drug Stress Trauma Syndrome (see page 67). [179]

8) When they do work, they tend to help mental, emotional and behavioral *symptoms* for only a few weeks or months. But by then the user is usually chemically dependant on the drug and will likely have a painful withdrawal experience if they try to stop taking it.

By contrast, **some** psychiatric drugs can help **some** people with mental, emotional and behavioral symptoms, although not usually for long. But they have limits, about which BigPharma and many clinicians do not usually warn when they recommend and prescribe psychiatric drugs.

Peter Breggin said, "It is difficult, if not impossible, to determine accurately the psychological condition of a person who is taking psychiatric drugs. There are too many complicating factors, including the drug's brain-disabling effect, the brain's compensatory reactions and the patient's psychological responses to taking the drug. I have evaluated many cases in which patients have deteriorated under the onslaught of multiple psychiatric drugs without the prescribing physicians attributing the patient's decline to drug toxicity. Instead, physicians [and the patient and their family] typically attribute their patients' worsening condition to 'mental illness' when in reality the patient is suffering from adverse drug reactions." [25]

Breggin's and others' work has reflected the sometime-missing conscience of psychiatry. For anyone who accepts help in the form of psychiatric drugs, realize that you are entering into an area that you *may regret* or *may not be able to stop*. Each drug has toxic effects that turn out to be as bad as or worse than the original complaint and often leads to more drugs to counter these toxic effects, which include drug withdrawal. Breggin spells this out in some detail in his comprehensive 2008 textbook. [25]

Figure 12.1 A Few of Many Reasons to Avoid Psychiatric Drugs

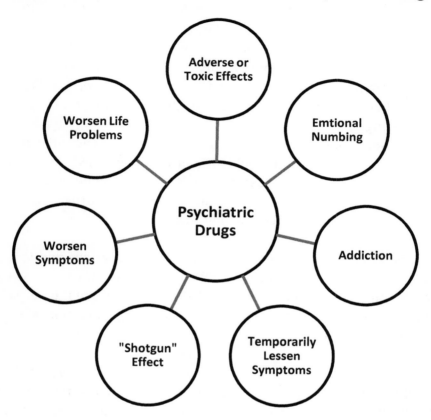

Stopping using psychiatric drugs successfully usually requires the person to initiate and maintain several actions long term. These actions include the following:

1) Begin and maintain a program of regular exercise and healthy nutrition, including taking high quality multi-vitamins daily. I and others suggest some nutritional *supplements* for you to take as well, described below.

2) If you experience bothersome fear, anxiety, panic, or insomnia, you can begin a pre-taper program to help settle you down enough to then be able to start the

tapering process. Details are explained by researcher and author James Harper in his book *How to Get off Psychiatric Drugs Safely* (Harper 2010). [72]

3) Learn healthy sleep habits and use sleep supplements (avoid taking common toxic sleeping pills such as Ambien, Lunesta, Sonata, Klonopin or other benzodiazapine sedatives), as shown in Chapter 15 on page 185.

4) Begin and maintain seeing a counselor or therapist if you grew up in a troubled family or have PTSD due to repeated hurts, losses and traumas; avoid seeing anyone who promotes your using psych drugs long term, or simply decline their drug suggestions.

This latter recovery work will help you name, grieve and let go of the emotional pain that psychiatric drugs temporarily relieved when you started them originally. These kinds of emotional pain may include fear, anxiety, depression, low energy, low self esteem, and difficulty sleeping.

Learning to tolerate emotional pain and *handle our conflicts* in a *healthy way* is key to preventing relapse. [188] Regular attendance at Adult Children of Alcoholics, Co-dependents Anonymous, Al-Anon or Emotions Anonymous meetings and trauma centered group therapy can facilitate all of the above.

When you have initiated and continued the above for several weeks, THEN you can begin to slowly taper off using your psychiatric drugs—one drug at a time. If you are taking more than one psych drug, *select which drug* you will *get off first*. For that selected drug try decreasing your total daily maintenance dose by 10% for the next two weeks. Then lower the dose by another 10% (now 20% of the total) for another two weeks. Continue decreasing the daily dose by 10% every two weeks in this way until you have stopped the drug, one drug at a time. Tapering involves trial and error. Use the supplements described below and in Breggin and/or Harper's book to help as you taper.

Find a physician with expertise in helping people taper from psychiatric drugs (described more below). The hardest drug to taper and stop is usually a benzodiazepine. Next most difficult are antipsychotics and antidepressants. Then opiates, stimulants, and finally anti-epilepsy drugs ("mood stabilizers").

SELECTING WHICH DRUG TO GET OFF FIRST

When a person wants to taper and stop two or more psychiatric drugs, there are two general ways to consider. The first way is that described by Harper in his book *How to Get off Psychiatric Drugs Safely.* Through his extensive research and assisting countless people in this regard, he has summarized the metabolic breakdown of each of some 39 psychiatric drugs based on their cytochrome P450 enzyme pathways, as shown in Table 12.4 on page 152. Using this information Harper has found that when a person has been taking two or more psych drugs at the same time for longer than a few weeks, it generally works best to begin tapering the drug first that uses the fewest shared P450 pathways. There may be *some exceptions* to this method, e.g., Effexor has only 2 such pathways, yet along with Paxil, in part due to its short half life, is usually the most difficult to stop. This is in contrast to Prozac which has 7 such pathways but is easier to stop, in part because of its longer half-life and availability in liquid form.

While I take this approach into account, I also use another one based on my knowledge of psychiatric drugs and my clinical experience. Because some drugs and drug categories are harder to taper and stop, I look at *how difficult* each may be to get off, as shown in Table 12.1 on page 147. But at the same time I also consider *how toxic* the drug and/or the lifestyle associated with getting and using the drug may be. For example, for someone who is taking any drug that is especially toxic or detrimental to their health, I may recommend tapering it first. This is especially true for *amphetamine stimulants*, which commonly cause nervous tics, hypertension, and aggravate heart problems—plus for some patients a toxic lifestyle of finding and buying these drugs on the always-dangerous "street." It is also true for *lithium*, causing neurological and systemic problems such as kidney and other organ damage, and *antipsychotics* causing a wide range of bothersome and detrimental toxic effects.

I also look at *how long* the patient has been taking a drug. If that duration has been for less than a month, I often suggest tapering and stopping that drug first within a few weeks.

In summary, these are among several factors that I consider:

1) The drug's P450 or other metabolic pathways,
2) How toxic each drug is in general and in an individual patient,
3) How easy it is to get off the drug, and,
4) How long they have taken it.

Regarding a dependence on **opiate** pain killer drugs (not classic psychiatric drugs, but still psychoactive and addicting), there is an effective way out. This way includes transitioning them onto using maintenance by taking a special long-acting opiate drug daily called "buprenorphine" (trade names Suboxone and Subutex), which usually stops opiate withdrawal symptoms and their seeking other opiates. I ask most of such patients to attend one of the Twelve Step Fellowships of Alcoholics Anonymous or Narcotics Anonymous at least weekly. Later, when ready, they can slowly taper using the above and selected supplements, plus clonidine as needed to take the edge off of opiate withdrawal.

Table 12.1 Stopping psychiatric drugs, with *increasing* order of difficulty

Drug Category	Comments
Anti-epileptics, aka "mood stabilizers" including lithium	Decrease dose slowly over several weeks to 3 months. These are generally sedative drugs, which often over-sedate. *Use supplement protocol below to assist in all these drug categories.*
Stimulants	Decrease dose slowly over several weeks to 3 months, or if need by 10% per 2 weeks or more. Use supplement protocol to assist.
Opiate pain killers	Transfer to buprenorphine, begin 12 Step work; taper when ready.
Antipsychotics & Antidepressants	Decrease total dose by 10% per 2 weeks or more, usually by trial & error. Hardest to stop are Effexor and Paxil. May need to switch ADPs to liquid form if available as Prozac & Paxil to lower dose more accurately & slowly
Benzodiazepines *usually hardest to stop*	Decrease total dose by 10% per 2 weeks or more, usually by trial & error. Hardest to stop are ones with short half lives, as Xanax, etc.

Many to most of my patients who are on psychiatric drugs have PTSD, which was usually not diagnosed and thereby usually mistreated with psychiatric drugs. So I also take this into consideration: many of their original psychiatric and psychological problems may actually be *signs and symptoms of their PTSD* and/or they may also be due to the *toxic effects of the psych drugs* they take, including withdrawal symptoms when they miss or skip a dose (Table A.3 page 203). Also important is whether the person has a healthy support system and is in an appropriate recovery program for their PTSD. I further describe drug withdrawal manifestations and dynamics in Tables A.2 through A.6 in the Appendix on pages 199 through 209.

EXPECTATIONS WHEN TAPERING & STOPPING PSYCH DRUGS

The experience of tapering and stopping psychiatric drugs is of course not pain free emotionally and physically. Be prepared to experience and endure mild to moderate levels of this pain. Even so, using the approach in this chapter and elsewhere in this book, and if time and interest, in Harper's, Breggin's, Lehmann's, Glenmullen's, or Hall's books (see references), there are ways to make getting off drugs easier.

For example, for fear or anxiety, one may use such aides as exercise, the EFT acupressure tapping technique,[192] and the supplements in Table 12.2. Using the supplements usually involves a trial and error approach. Try the tart cherry concentrate first. If no positive results, add a dose of passion flower, 5HTP, l-theanine, or GABA, one at a time. If still no results, one can try increasing the *dose* of what was added, or adding another one from this group.

Four of the supplements in the lower section of Table 12.2 should be taken daily and long-term. These include: omega 3 fatty acids and quality multi vitamins (the vitamins ideally with each meal). Also, a balanced food intake that includes a protein source that keeps us focusing and functioning. Harper recommends also using a whey protein concentrate supplement. While Harper recommends it, I have little experience using beta 1,3-D glucan.

This tapering will likely take several to many months for each different psych drug, for which the attitude of patience and persistence will provide a distinct advantage. Do not try to rush the process. Harper also recommends that if there is bothersome fear or anxiety, agitation or insomnia (or you want to taper an antipsychotic)—before the tapering has begun that the person begin a pre-tapering process by using especially the tart cherry concentrate, passion flower extract, beta 1, 3-D glucan, and whey protein concentrate. I usually advise adding the daily supplements and vitamins mentioned in the above paragraph. Also for pre-tapering use the sleep hygiene and supplement program described in the chapter on sleep. For details in pre-tapering, see chapters 6, 9 and 10 in Harper's book, also available online at www.TheRoadBack.org.

KEEPING A DAILY JOURNAL

Another aid will be to print out a daily journal in the form of a chart that monitors and describes how you are functioning in each of your key areas, as shown in Table 12.3. In this chart rate your experience in each life area on a scale from 1 to 10 by daily writing a 1 for the worst you have felt or can feel or function, and a 10 for the best. Take a copy of this chart that you keep up-to-date when you meet with your clinician who is helping you with this tapering process. To find such a clinician will likely take a lot of looking and asking around. If you can find a holistically oriented physician or psychiatrist—not an easy task—who will be willing to help you get off one or more of these drugs *and not give you more psych drugs*, you will be fortunate. If any clinicians try to prescribe any more psychiatric drugs (except buspirone &/or phenytoin), decline them and keep them focused on the taper. If they don't, you can leave.

*   *   *

If living as one who is mentally ill (crazy, somehow defective, or other shameful terms) and taking psychiatric drugs has been and is now working for you to give you what you think is a healthy whole life, I wish you the best. Then you may not need this chapter right now. But if continuing to take the drug(s) long-term does not work for you, I invite you to reconsider my observations.

Table 12.2. Supplements to help taper & stop psychiatric drugs

Supplement	Dose	Comment
Tart cherry concentrate	1 tsp in ½ glass H2O	Anti-anxiety effect in 15 minutes, lasts about 4 hrs. Can take every 2 hours if needed.
Passion flower extract	200-400 mg	Herbal anti-anxiety & sedative agent
5 HTP	100 to 300 mg	Amino acid anti-anxiety & sedative agent
l-theanine	100 mg or more	Amino acid anti-anxiety agent; may potentiate melatonin effect; may help some with OCD
GABA	100 mg or more	Amino acid anti-anxiety agent & sleep aid. GABA = gamma-aminobutyric acid
Quality vitamins	With each meal	Esp. Bs (1,3,6 & 12), folic acid, & C help absorption & metabolism of all above
Omega 3s	1 tsp daily	Helps brain & nervous system, needs vitamin E
dl - phenylalanine	½-1 gm	May help most difficult drug WD; avoid after 3 pm
Whey protein isolate	1 tsp+ in any liquid daily	Helps benefit of quality protein intake, needed esp. in psych drug withdrawal & for vegetarians
Inulin	5 grams/day	Chicory root fiber, natural pre-biotic helping calcium absorption & healthier colon function
beta 1,3-D glucan	100 mg empty stomach/day	Helps raise interleukin 2 & 6 blood level for increased immune system strength

Charles L. Whitfield, M.D.

Table 12.3 Daily Functioning Log

NAME _____ DATE_____

RATE 1-10 WHERE APPROPRIATE

1= NORMAL OR GOOD 10 = WORST EVER

Area or Action	Day 1	Day 2	Day 3	Day 4	Day 5	Day 6	Day 7
Mood							
Anxiety							
Energy							
Ability to focus							
Fatigue							
Pains							
Appetite							
Exercise							
Nausea							
Muscle Twitching							
Sleep							
Meditation Prayer							
Journaling Meetings							
Overall functioning							

Area or Action	Day 1	Day 2	Day 3	Day 4	Day 5	Day 6	Day 7
Drugs & doses taken & when							
Supple-ments taken							
Cherry							

Table 12.4 P450 enzyme pathways for drug metabolism (expanded from Harper 2005)

Antidepressant	IA2	2C19	2C9	2D6	3A
Prozac *	X	X	X	X	X
Zoloft *	X	X	X	X	X
Luvox *	X	X	X	X	X
Remeron	X	X	X	X	X
Paxil *	X	X	X	X	
Anafranil	X	X		X	X
Tofranil *	X	X		X	X
Wellbutrin *	X		X	X	X
Elavil *	X	X		X	
Effexor				X	X
Lexapro		X		X	
Celexa		X		X	
Cymbalta	X			X	
Pamelor				X	X
Trazodone				X	X

Table 12.4. P450 enzyme pathways for drug metabolism

(expanded from Harper 2005)...continued

Antipsychotic	IA2	2C19	2C9	2D6	3A
Clozaril *	X	X	X	X	X
Abilify				X	X
Geodon *	X				X
Haldol *	X			X	
Risperdal *				X	X
Zyprexa *	X			X	
Seroquel *					X
Others					
Depakote *	X	X	X		X
Valium/Xanax *		X			X
Klonopin *					X
Ambien	X		X		X
Strattera		X		X	

All are trade names but **trazodone**.

* Have more pathways: **Elavil** - UGT1 A4, UGT1 A3, P-gp; **Luvox** - 2B6, P-gp, intestinal 3A; **Paxil** & **Prozac** - 2B6, P-gp; **Tofranil** - UGT1A4, 3, P-gp; **Wellbutrin** - 2E1, 2A6, 2B6; **Zoloft** - UGT2B7, UGT1A4, P-gp, 2B6; **Clozaril** - FMO, UGT1A4, UGT1A3; **Geodon** - aldehyde oxidase substrate; **Haldol** - glucuronidation, Pgp; **Risperdal** - P-gp, renal extraction; **Seroquel** - glucuronidation, P-gp, intestinal 3A, epoxide by quetiapine; **Zyprexa** - glucuronidation, FMO, UGT1A4; **BuSpar** [usually no withdrawal symptoms]- intestinal 3A, 2D6; **Depakote** - UGT2B7, UGT1A6, UGT1A9, UGT2B15, UGT1A4, UGT1A3; **Valium** - 2B6, UGT2B7, intestinal 3A; **Zanax** - hepatic 3A; **Concerta** & **Ritalin** glucuronidation.

The Stimulants all have 2D6 (**Adderall, Dextrostat, Ritalin, Concerta**-latter 2 also have glucuronidation pathway).

13 Remembering & Processing Trauma

Remembering our trauma mentally and experientially is a key to healing from its painful effects. Being labeled with "mental illness" or a "mental disorder" and taking psychiatric drugs usually numbs or distracts us from this crucial remembering and healing, leaving us dissociated from our real self and its crucial inner life. *Dissociation* is a basic term that we can use to help us understand trauma and its effects. Understanding what it is and its dynamics is a key to recognizing what happened and how to heal from the painful effects of trauma. Here I will get a bit technical, so bear with me.

DISSOCIATION

People who have experienced abuse or trauma frequently report: "I went numb," "I just wasn't there," or "I left my body." To dissociate means to *separate*. Dissociation is a process whereby information—incoming, stored or outgoing—is actively *blocked* or *deflected* from our full awareness and integration (i.e., healthy realizing, understanding and handling). Clinical and research psychiatrist David Spiegel further defined dissociation as being ". . . analogous to working in one directory of a computer without being able to access the main menu, indicating the presence of other directories and without path commands enabling the directory to find information needed from another directory. The presence of the material in one directory makes the computer act as though the other material does not exist." [150] Psychologist Frank Leavitt defines dissociation as losing our awareness and connections to our experience partially or fully. [94,174] It happens when we "tune out," "space out," or forget an experience.

Charles L. Whitfield, M.D.

We can dissociate across a spectrum of being in *healthy trance states* to defending against *emotional* pain to having PTSD and/or a *dissociative disorder,* as shown in Figure 13.1.

Figure 13.1. Spectrum of Dissociation [174]

Healthy Dissociation		"Grey Zone"		Unhealthy Dissociation	
Healthy Trance States	Defending Against the Pain of Being Abused as a Child	Defending Against the Pain of Being Abused as an Adult	PTSD	Dissociative Disorder (DD)	Dissociative Identity Disorder (MPD)

Dissociation is a *protective* and *useful* survival defense for growing up in an unhealthy family and world. When we are being mistreated or abused, dissociating allows us to separate from our awareness of our inner life, especially our painful feelings and thoughts. *Here* it serves a *useful* purpose. But after we grow up and leave that family, to dissociate frequently from all pain may no longer be necessary or particularly useful, especially if we are now around safe or safer people. But what was an adaptive and useful skill in defending against the pain of childhood abuse may continue into adulthood as a maladaptive habit. Dissociation may be *maladaptive* in two ways. First, as just mentioned, the adult pain-dissociator who has left the abusive environment of home and neighborhood may now live in a safe environment, yet they may continue to dissociate unnecessarily, thus hampering their interactions and relationships. Or second, they may remain in their abusive environment or move into another one, and while their ability to dissociate may still be useful, it may block their ability to access their **inner life** accurately and appropriately (see Figure 13.2). In either of these situations, the person may age-regress frequently, which can also rob them of their ability to feel confident and in charge of their life and enjoy it. Age regression is

155

a dissociative state, and many of the principles for its healing apply for many of the other varieties of dissociation, as I describe in *A Gift to Myself* and *Boundaries and Relationships*. Most psych drugs also block our ability to access our inner life—yet another toxic effect—via a kind of chemical dissociation.

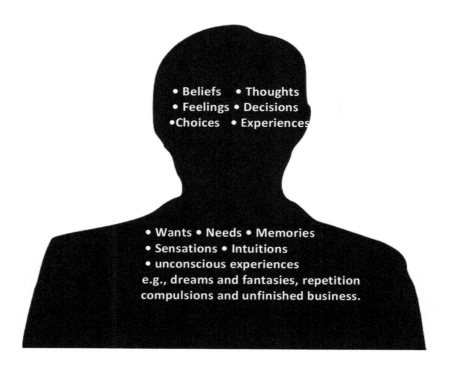

Figure 13.2 My Inner Life

As adults, if we continue to dissociate, we may feel as though we have lost the "point of contact" with our inner and outer reality. We often feel "out of touch," with the present moment, "artificial," or as though we are "play acting." As we heal we take control of the mechanism of dissociating and become more in touch with our authentic inner life in the present moment.

FOUR AREAS OF DISSOCIATION

We may dissociate our awareness and experience in any of several of our life areas—the physical, mental, emotional and spiritual. The following include some examples:

Physical: Out-of-body experience, psychogenic or hysterical anesthesia or paralysis, drug intoxication – *especially* when we take *psychiatric drugs*, alcohol or other drugs, physical self harm, violence to another, overeating, purging or starving.

Mental: Separating or distancing from one or more inner-life components, such as our beliefs, thoughts and memories; fantasizing, intellectualizing; "splitting off."

Emotional: Separating from our feelings, whether painful or joyful, "numbing out," smiling or laughing at pain, "poker face" or a mask, age-regressing.

Spiritual: All of the above, as exemplified by age-regression, plus feeling separated from others and the God of our understanding.

We may dissociate in any one or more of these areas in a healthy or an unhealthy way. We may also dissociate as an individual, or collectively as a group. Individuals may dissociate frequently, e.g., when they *mean*, "I get angry," but instead, they *say* "*You* get angry" or "*One* gets angry." An example of collective dissociation is calling something by another name, such as when we call homelessness "displaced person status," or when we call fear "anxiety," and call sadness or grief "depression."

Healthy trance states like daydreaming, writing a song or poem, listening to a symphony, or even a jogger's high, are common.

DISSOCIATIVE DISORDERS

Also common is the psychological defense of dissociation in reaction to the stress and traumas of everyday life. Actual *disorders* of dissociation are relatively common (as in dissociative amnesia) to rare (dissociative fugue). Here I also describe their salient characteristics. **Dissociative amnesia** is relatively common among survivors of trauma—hence its alternative name of ***traumatic* amnesia**. As of 1999 sixty-eight data based studies showed that about a third of CSA (child sexual abuse) survivors *completely* forget long-term that they were sexually abused, while another third always remember it, with the middle third having *partial* amnesia for the trauma. [35,36,168,172]

Dissociative identity disorder (DID, also called multiple personality disorder wherein a person displays multiple distinct identities or personalities known as "alters," each with its own pattern of perceiving and interacting with the environment) and the other dissociative disorders (DDs) frequently involve some degree of dissociative amnesia. [146] I give 3 case history examples and then address trauma memory further at the end of this chapter.

After 19 years of media publicity about a claimed "false memory syndrome"—which tried through pseudoscience to deny the reality of dissociative or traumatic amnesia—there has been no data based study showing the existence of anything like a "false memory syndrome." It appears that the term was made up in 1992 by an organized group of accused (by their own adult children) and convicted child molesters that called itself the false memory syndrome foundation. Most aware clinicians have always viewed this claim as part of their denial system and overall a hoax. A problem was that many in the media and some unaware in the public believed it. [35,36,168,172]

HISTORY 13.1

Amy was a forty-four-year-old single, recovering alcoholic woman with dissociative identity disorder . She was referred to me by a colleague for work on healing the effects of her severe childhood trauma. When I first saw her she knew that she had DID, with about six "alter" personalities, but she knew little about them. As I worked with her over time in individual and group therapy, I noted that she had great difficulty identifying and expressing her feelings. She had only fragmentary memories about the severe abuse and neglect that she suffered as a child. However, when her alter personalities surfaced they were better able to name and express her feelings and describe her traumatic memories. When she became stressed or sleep-deprived, she frequently "switched," as an alter personality would assume her identity, and this experience aggravated her stress level such that she drank, missed work, and finally lost her job.

Early in the course of her recovery, she relapsed into alcoholic drinking several more times, necessitating four hospitalizations. She eventually strengthened her alcoholism recovery program and began to stabilize, and then found a job where she could support herself. In individual and group therapy, over time she began slowly to get to know her alters and, more importantly, to feel, own and express her feelings more authentically. She spent the next four years in the active stage of grief work, feeling and expressing the un-grieved pain of her severe childhood trauma and neglect. She ultimately switched less often and is now approaching a state of "integration," wherein she is able to live as and from her true self (also called the "core" personality by DID clinical researchers and authors).

Amy's story illustrates the difficulty that people with DID experience as they try to heal. [146] Before she could enter into a

Stage Two full-recovery program, she had to stabilize her almost chaotic life, which was aggravated by her flooding memories of the trauma and frequent alcoholic relapses wherein she tried to lessen her pain. As with most people with DID, she had several other (also called co-morbid) disorders, including alcoholism, "depression" and PTSD. My experience is that people with dissociative disorders represent an extreme end of the effects of trauma and that they usually require more time and patience to recover. Amy has now been active and successful in her trauma-focused recovery work for over six years.

HISTORY 13.2

Tony was a forty-six-year-old divorced dentist who had the disorder called *dissociative fugue* since he was a young man. He came for assistance with trying to heal from a life of frustration and pain. He had to stop practicing dentistry because of disability from his dissociative fugue and severe PTSD. He was sexually and psychologically abused by his mother after having been abandoned by his father when he was two years old. He had great difficulty expressing his feelings in both individual and group therapy. After three years of recovery work, he went to work for a dental clinic that provided services for a low-income neighborhood. Gradually his fugue states, in which he unpredictably dissociated and traveled, only to awaken and not remember what he had done, decreased. He is now in his fifth year of work on his recovery and is moderately improved from his debilitating symptoms.

Both Amy and Tony's histories show how long and painful the process of recovery is for many people with dissociative disorders. Their recovery is commonly aggravated by other life problems, such as "depression," addictions and PTSD. Most of the people with DID and many with the other dissociative disorders over time have seen several health professionals, many of whom have paid little attention to their childhood trauma issues. They have commonly

160

lost jobs, become disabled and so financially strapped that they have difficulty paying for their treatment. These disorders are toward the far end of the spectrum of severity regarding the effects of trauma, approaching those with debilitating schizophrenia, which I discuss in Chapters 17 and 18 of *The Truth about Mental Illness* and with John Read and colleagues in a recent comprehensive article linking it to a trauma history. [128]

When we dissociate in a *healthy* way, we may focus our awareness on only one or two areas of our experience. Or we may shift, and scan many areas. Dissociation is thus a great facility and skill through which we may explore and experience parts of our life. *Unhealthy* dissociation can be differentiated from the healthy kind by 1) a significant alteration in a person's sense of *identity*, as seen in DID and fugue states—as well as in the common *numbed* dissociation of our true self when we let our false self run our life—and by 2) a partial or complete loss of *memory* for a traumatic event [151,158] and by 3) the other maladaptive kind of dissociation, including the spellbinding effect of psychiatric drugs (page 209 in the Appendix).

In all my years of practice, I have never seen a person with a dissociative disorder who grew up in a healthy family. Nearly all also have PTSD. These dissociative disorders, along with PTSD and anxiety disorders, appear to be mostly disorders of *fear*. Each of these people grew up in a dysfunctional family that usually repeatedly shamed and threatened them, leaving the child in a continuous state of post-traumatic fear that manifested as either *hyper-stimulation, hyperactivity,* or a feeling of *numbness,* or an alternating of these.

With no healthy models to teach us otherwise and no safe people or places to share and process our inner and outer life, and because these are often so painful or confusing, we may split off any of these components of our experience and bury them deep within the unconscious part of our psyche. This is similar to what I have referred to as "The Child or True Self going into hiding" (as shown on page 120). This dissociation, separation or splitting off of one or more of these components may come about in any pattern or sequence. A common pattern is when a person *cognitively* (mentally) *remembers* aspects of a traumatic experience but dissociates from their associated *feelings*, sensations or images for a long time, as the following history illustrates.

HISTORY 13.3

At age thirty, Susan came for counseling because she had recently felt a repulsion for her five-year-old son and had begun to reject him physically and emotionally. After several counseling sessions she began to remember that her mother had treated her the same way when she was five, although more severely. It was at this age when she had realized that her mother was very disturbed. While she had always *cognitively* remembered that she had been sexually abused by a baby-sitter at age six and by her grandfather at age nine, she had *forgotten her painful emotions* that were *attached* to the *experience* of being molested. While talking about it with her therapist, her painful feelings gradually returned. She then remembered telling her mother about it immediately after having been molested by her grandfather (her mother's father), and her mother's dissociating and completely ignoring her. At that time, Susan realized that he had likely molested her mother as a child also. When she was thirty she told her aunt about it, who believed her and validated her experience. After expressing her story and her pain, she was able to grieve the trauma that she had not been able to before. Her feeling of repulsion or her son then gradually disappeared.

Susan's experience is an example of a frequent pattern of dissociation after trauma that is not allowed to be processed when it happened. It shows how, even in those who have always cognitively remembered trauma, that, having dissociated from the hurt, they may still have un-grieved pain to experience and work through. During her process of remembering and grieving, she said, "It was as though my memories were under a stairway in the dark recesses of my mind. A part of me always knew they were there, but I never wanted to shine the light on them." While she was able to resolve her presenting complaint symptoms in four months of weekly psychotherapy, three years later she continues to work on her residual associated pain and core issues, and her functioning as an individual, wife and mother show clear improvement.

TRAUMA MEMORIES ARE CORRECT IN ESSENCE

Since ordinary memory is often inaccurate, some critics have rightly expressed concern about the possibility that retrospective reports based on our memory of childhood trauma could also be inaccurate. To address this concern, several independent researchers looked at this question from different perspectives and by using different research methods over a 17-year span from 1985 to 2002. I found nine examples of these investigations. Six were data based studies on 6,546 people and three were extensive reviews of the current research literature available from 1998 through 2002. As summarized in Table 13.1 on the next 2 pages, these examples show that not only is trauma memory different than ordinary memory, but it is also generally accurate in its essence, i.e., in this case that the childhood **trauma actually occurred**. These reports from diverse authors and study samples show that 1) trauma memory is generally accurate and 2) trauma memory data from retrospective studies is usually reliable.

Table 13.1. Self-Reporting and Remembering Accuracy

Year/Author	Study Characteristics	Findings among trauma survivors
1985 Robins et al.	52 alcoholics or depressives 39 controls	Memories of child environment experience mostly valid 1
1988 Berger et al.	Study 1: 4,695 college students, Study 2: 34 social service managed teens	12% were physically injured by parent, yet only 2.9% said they were abused 2
1993 Brewin et al.	Extensive review of retrospective report accuracy	Central features of trauma memories are likely to be reasonably accurate 3
1997 Bifulco et al.	87 twin sister pairs evaluated	High cross-corroboration of trauma memories 4
1998 Brown et al.	Extensive review & analysis of literature on dissociative amnesia & critical literature	All 68 reports that studied CSA memory found DA** in about 1/3 of subjects 5
2000 Fergusson et al. Prospective	1,265 children followed 21 years from birth	Significant false negative reports about trauma 6
2001 Richter & Eisermann	220 psych inpatients	Memories of parenting were generally consistent & credible 7
2001 Whitfield et al.	Special volume on misinformation spread by CSA memory critics (incl. accused & convicted child molester groups)	Extensive reviews showed no data based evidence for a "false memory syndrome" 8
2002 Wilsnack et al.	154 CSA women, structured interview, 37 with dis. amnesia	Only 3 of 37 remembered with help of a clinician 9
Summary: 1985–2002 9 Reports	**6 Studies (on 6,546 people) & 3 Literature Reviews (of numerous reports)**	**Conclusion: 10 Trauma memory is generally accurate (when positive)**

...of Childhood Trauma: 9 Example Studies or Reviews

Other Findings	*Comments*
1 A significant number had true memories	Psychiatric disorders did not appear to bias reports
2 *Under-reporting* of trauma is *common*	Most abused failed to label themselves as having been abused
3 Confirming reports are given more weight than negative ones	Linking trauma memories to current pain is helpful
4 Childhood trauma memories are mostly valid	A strong twin study result
5 Most of the 63 cited critical reports did not examine memory for CSA	Dissociative amnesia is a real and common phenomenon among CSA survivors
6 Single negative reports are unreliable	Numerous effects of trauma found
7 Depressed patients	High stability of memories
8 Memory critics often use a contrived denial system on trauma memory	Examples given and discussed of an extensive disinformation campaign by accused child molesters
9 Clinician-assisted recall is rare	Childhood sexual abuse memories are mostly valid
10 Some critics' bias may be substantial	**Retrospective trauma memory data are usually reliable**

* For ethical and humanistic reasons, prospective studies cannot be conducted in CSA and other childhood traumas. Even so, when researchers find already-existing abused populations to evaluate and follow, they can do so ethically, as these reports have shown, and all of them found dissociative (traumatic) amnesia to occur in a substantial percentage of CSA survivors (Brown et al. 1998). **DA = dissociative amnesia; CSA = child sexual abuse.

These findings have also been substantiated by over 300 published studies on trauma effects, including over 30 prospective studies that have replicated the same results. This is in contrast to the disinformation promoted by "false memory" advocates, who in 19 years of their claims since 1992 — as mentioned above — have not produced any published convincing evidence of the existence of a "false memory syndrome" for child sexual abuse or other traumas.

RECOVERY PRINCIPLES

Addressing dissociation involves becoming more aware of it when it happens to us. A starting point is to learn about a common form of dissociation called *age-regression,* and what it is and how to handle it. I describe age-regression in some detail in my books *A Gift to Myself* (page 181) and *Memory and Abuse* (page 155). Healthy and unhealthy dissociation happens throughout the long process of recovery from any of the various effects of trauma. When it occurs, attending to each of these effects by healthy expression of our inner-life with safe people will usually increase the chance for an earlier recovery.

As is true for most of the other disorders or life problems that are aggravated or caused by trauma, using a stage-oriented approach is most helpful, as I describe in Table 14.1 on page 174 in the next chapter. A key Stage One recovery principle for DID is to recognize and name it, and then stabilize from its disruptive effects. In Stage Two we do the trauma work directly by the long process of *uncovering, remembering* and *naming* our traumas and then grieving about their hurtful effects. Each time that we work through a memory or a painful issue, we tend to get stronger. Many recovery aids are useful in healing. Of these, individual and group therapy are especially helpful.

PROCESSING DISSOCIATED MEMORIES

People in recovery from dissociative and other "mental disorders" tend to have a broad range of past and ongoing emotional and physical pain, such as intrusive post-traumatic stress symptoms, dissociative symptoms, and painful psycho-physiological (mind-body) reactivity. True recovered memories are typically accompanied by significant emotional distress.

Recent research has addressed the natural history of recovered memories, which my colleagues Dan Brown, Alan Scheflin and I have described in some detail. [35] Memory of the trauma usually persists *both* as an overt, verbal or explicit narrative memory *and* a hidden, covert, implicit behavioral and somatic (body) memory. While these clinical findings often evolve in the order shown in Figure 13.3 below, they may also *evolve* in a *different sequence.* Working through these phases over time in the process of recovering the narrative memory strengthens recovery by *decreasing dissociation* and leading to a sense of *mastery over* the traumatic experience and effects. [35]

SYMPTOMS OFTEN GET "WORSE" BEFORE THEY GET BETTER

Clinical and research psychologists Diana Elliott and John Briere evaluated 113 adults who had been sexually abused as children and compared them with 385 controls (those with no history of CSA). They found that those with the *most recent* recovered memories of the traumas were the most symptomatic (i.e., they were in the most emotional, relationship and behavioral pain) when compared with those who had a *longer memory* of the abuse and those who had *always remembered* the abuse, and especially when compared to the *controls,* [51] (Figure A.1 on page 226). Other clinicians and I have observed these findings in countless CSA survivors who we have assisted as they healed. This is important

Figure 13.3. The Natural History of the Evolution of Memory Recovery in Childhood Sexual Abuse
(expanded from Brown, Scheflin & Whitfield 1999)*

Clinical Findings** Usually occur in ↓ this sequence 1 through 7	Example References
1. Transference re-enactments (in &/or out of therapy/recovery)*** ↓	Burgess et al. 1995; Terr 1994; Laplanche & Pontalis, 1973
2. Somatic & psychological symptoms ↓	Cameron 1996; van der Kolk & Fisler 1995; Pomerantz 1999
3. Flashbacks, abreactions & age regressions ↓	above plus: Roe & Schwartz 1996; Kristiansen et al.,1995; Whitfield 1995,1997,1998
4. Dreams & nightmares ↓	Whitfield 1995,1997, 1998; Kristiansen et al. 1995
5. Fragmented narrative memory (triggered by reminder events)	Cameron 1996; Kristiansen et al. 1995; van der Kolk & Fisler 1995
6. Obsessive thoughts of trauma ↓	Terr 1994
7. Organized narrative memory - with or without healing & recovery	van der Kolk & Fisler 1995 (none showed initial return of memory as narrative memory, which tended to occur last)

* Working through these stages as they occurred decreased dissociation and led to a sense of mastery over the trauma and its effects.

** Clinical findings are from Davies & Frawley 1994, Whitfield 1995, 1997, 1998, 2004 and other cited references, and all may be manifestations of PTSD. *Triggering events* such as recurrent traumas or reminders of them commonly initiate these kinds of memory (Whitfield, 1995b). Over the extended time of healing and recovery these clinical findings tend to progress from being vague to clearer. *** These clinical findings may occur in different sequences, e.g., #2 may be the initial experience, then skip to #5, and then continue as #6 and #7.

information, since the trauma survivor and the person's family and friends often erroneously believe that the survivor is mentally ill and/or is "making up" the trauma memory. They often need to be reassured that *neither* is true. Rather, their *symptoms* and *concerns* are *part of the natural history of recovery from trauma.* [51,36,168]

In recovery, as we heal in the company of safe people, we can begin to *recognize* when we are dissociating (same as age regressing). If we are in group or individual therapy, the others can mirror or tell us what they see and hear. Other therapy group members can also describe what is coming up for them from their inner lives as we tell our stories and describe how we are feeling. We can also experiment with *deliberately* trying to *dissociate.* Bringing what was formerly unconscious into our conscious awareness can be empowering. As we dissociate—that is, alter our state of consciousness by separating or distancing from our full awareness—we can practice increasing or decreasing the clarity of our experience. We can thereby gain more awareness and control over what once may have felt was out of control for us. Identifying which *people* or *situations* may *trigger* the experiences of dissociation is also useful. Then we can begin to *set healthy boundaries* and *limits* when we are around them so that they will not continue to hurt us. [167]

When we dissociate, we involuntarily alter our state of consciousness. The person who can move spontaneously from one state of consciousness to another can have several advantages. One is that in recovery they may eventually be able to access their unconscious feelings and other inner life material more easily. And they can go in and out of therapeutic trance more easily. While fear is still often a block for some, they may be able to make more constructive use of experiential techniques in their recovery.

In the next chapter I continue with a summary of the essential parts of the recovery process.

14 Recovery Process & Core Issues

Throughout this book I have commented on various aspects of real and effective treatment, and I describe the recovery process in some detail in my books *Healing the Child Within*, *A Gift to Myself, Boundaries and Relationships, Memory and Abuse* and *The Truth About Depression.*[24]

Accurate information is golden. Perhaps the first bit of information that you may have noticed is that your pain (emotional, behavioral and relationship-related) does *not* mean that you are mentally ill. You may have been given a wrong diagnosis and a wrong treatment. Your pain and suffering are most likely simply (or perhaps at times complexly) due to the • effects of the repeated and many traumas you have experienced *combined* with • how you know and choose to handle your conflicts day-to-day. How you handle your conflicts day-to-day may be related to living from your ego instead of your real self and any accompanying unhealed core recovery issues. [177,178]

Having read this far you may have begun to identify that you may have experienced some hurtful trauma and that it may have resulted in some effects and difficulties for you throughout your life. This insight can open the door to an eventually more peaceful life. And this insight usually comes from reframing the past mis-information that you were mentally ill into the new information

---

[24] **Note:** Other clinicians have described trauma recovery in their good books (examples include: Herman 1992, Davies and Frawley 1994, Briere 1996, Courtois 1998, Chu 1998, McCann and Pearlman 1990, Cashdan 1988, Gold 2000, Wilson et al. 2001, Karon 1981 and Kluft 1993, Courtois, Ford, van der Kolk, Herman 2010).

that your pain is but a manifestation of the *effects of your life traumas* and *how you handle adversities*. This can be powerful information. Identifying and *naming things accurately* is personal power, which is among several things that you can do to facilitate your healing over time. [164,165]

You may now suspect or even know that you are not crazy. You are not mentally ill. Instead, you may be just traumatized or wounded and have PTSD. If you were mistreated with toxic psychiatric drugs they may *not* have helped you enough or at all, and they may have made you worse. This kind of information was and is kept seemingly well hidden by the Bigs and other authority figures. **Now you know it**. With all of this information you may now be ready and able to make yourself a recovery plan that addresses your problems accurately and directly.

THE 10 RECOVERY PRINCIPLES

The focus of healing is on several tasks, which I described in *Healing the Child Within* 25 years ago. To rediscover our true or real self and heal our Child Within (with caps or not), we can begin a process that involves the following four actions of the 10 recovery principles.

1) Discover and practice being our **real self** or **child within**.
2) Identify our ongoing physical, mental-emotional and spiritual **needs**. Practice getting these needs met with safe and supportive people.
3) Identify, re-experience and **grieve** the pain of our ungrieved losses or traumas in the presence of safe and supportive people.
4) Identify and work through our **core** recovery **issues** (briefly described below, elsewhere [164,165,167,] and in detail in my book *Wisdom to Know the Difference*: Core Issues in Relationships, Recovery and Living). [188]

171

These 4 actions are closely related, although not listed in any particular order. Working on them, and thereby healing our Child Within, generally occurs in a circular fashion, with work and discovery in one area a link to another area.

Other key and related tasks include:
5) setting healthy **boundaries** and limits, 6) learning to **identify** and **work through day-to-day conflict** often associated with
7) **age-regression** and how to handle it, and 8) learning to **tolerate emotional pain** without self-medicating. I describe these in some detail in *Boundaries and Relationships* and *A Gift to Myself*. I have already addressed some important features of remembering our traumas. Having 9) **patience** and being **persistent** also help. Finally, learn about 10) the **stages of recovery**, which I describe after the next section on recovery aids.

THE 5 RECOVERY AIDS

These 5 recovery aids give us structure, guidance and support to accomplish these 10 principles.

Therapy or counseling: Find a trauma-recovery savvy therapist and early-on briefly interview them about what is in *this book* and in *Healing the Child Within*. If they push the idea that you are mentally ill of any variety (excluding PTSD, which is not a mental illness, but can feel and look like one to the uninformed) and if they recommend psych drugs, politely thank them for their opinion and exit their premises. Exception: if they suggest that you continue on the drug(s) *while* they slowly assist or support you *tapering* them. Individual &/or group therapy are key recovery aids.

Twelve Step Fellowship work and assistance: at CoDA (Co-dependents Anonymous), ACA (Adult Children of Alcoholics [& Trauma]), EA (Emotions Anonymous), Al-Anon (for family &

friends of alcoholics or drug dependents). Go to each meeting a few minutes early and stay 10 minutes after it to hear others' conversation. Eventually get a sponsor to assist you in working their Twelve suggested Steps over time.

Bibliotherapy: Read accurate and selected recovery information, which is also called *bibliotherapy*. Good books to start with are *Healing the Child Within* and *A Gift to Myself.* After reading those, I recommend *Boundaries and Relationships* and *Wisdom to Know the Difference.* If you may have problems remembering your traumas, review Chapter 13 on page 154, and consider looking at *Memory and Abuse.*

Personal Recovery Plan*: Make your own Recovery Plan as* described in either *A Gift to Myself* or *My Recovery: A Personal Plan for Healing.* If you need help, ask your therapist or sponsor. The ACA workbook can help.

No psychiatric drugs: As others and I describe, these don't work well—if at all—and they are toxic and mind numbing (Figure 14.1 on page 182 below). If you are currently taking any of them, consider reading or rereading Chapter 12 above on stopping them.

THE STAGES OF RECOVERY

While all acute injuries need some time to heal, *chronic* ones such as PTSD and the like tend to *take more time.* [164,165]

STAGE ZERO

Stage Zero is active illness, and here recovery has not yet begun. It is manifested by the presence of any active disorder, such as a mental or physical one, including depression, an addiction or any other problem. In this stage, you see both symptoms and signs and other *effects of whatever caused* the illness. This active illness may be acute, recurring or chronic. Without recovery, it may continue indefinitely—unless the person becomes somehow motivated to begin a Stage One effort. At Stage Zero, recovery has not yet started, as shown in Table 14.1.

Table 14.1. Recovery and Duration According to Stages

Recovery Stage	Condition	Focus of Recovery	Approximate Duration
3	Human/spiritual	Spirituality	Ongoing
2	Past trauma effects	Trauma-specific Recovery program	3–5+ years
1	Stage 0 disorder	Basic illness, full recovery program	Months to 3 years
0	Active illness	Usually none	Indefinite

* Note that this table reads from bottom to top

STAGE ONE

Coming to treatment for any mental or physical disorder is the beginning of Stage One. It involves participating in a full recovery program to assist in healing the Stage Zero disorder. It is the standard kind of process that we most commonly consider as conventional psychiatric or medical "treatment." If you are diabetic, you treat the diabetes by watching your diet, exercising, taking insulin and so forth. If you had "depression," you would often simply be prescribed an antidepressant drug, with little or no other investigation or intervention. Depending on the person and the problem, such a partial recovery program may be less likely to be as successful as a more complete regimen, which includes Stage Two. Stage One is the usual conventional, superficial treatment of mental disorders by using drugs alone. But that limited approach often does not work well. That is because most Stage One people usually come in with a presenting problem or concern that is actually the effect of the repeated trauma.

Promoted by the drug and managed care industries for at least the last thirty years, drug treatment is usually strongly recommended and prescribed for "depression" and most other presenting complaints that may remotely resemble a "mental disorder." [83] Unfortunately, this limited approach constitutes the bulk of their Stage One treatment today. Besides receiving drugs, a minority of people may get some brief counseling as well (if they are lucky enough to find a helping professional who recommends it—and if their managed care insurance company approves it). But that counseling is too often focused on only their current concerns, and seldom on past trauma effects. Brief therapy can help, depending on how much healing work is accomplished. Eventually, people may discover or awaken to having had an experience of trauma in their childhood and/or adulthood, and begin to connect it to their having subsequent mental and emotional pain.

STAGE TWO

The typical motivation for beginning Stage One recovery is hurting too much—emotional pain, physical pain or debilitating disease. But eventually, somewhere during, or more often after, Stage One recovery, people may realize that they are still hurting. They realize that whatever they have done before hasn't worked as well as they had hoped—that the Stage One approach alone didn't help them enough. So they might then be more open to exploring other alternatives. That is where they can begin a more substantial healing—if they are lucky enough to find a helping professional who knows Stage Two work.

Stage Two recovery involves healing the effects of repeated childhood and later trauma, including working through related core issues. Once a person has a stable and solid Stage One

175

recovery—one that has lasted for at least a few months to a year or longer—it may be time to consider looking into some of these Stage Two issues. Some mental disorders, especially those such as addictions (which commonly aggravate depression and anxiety), some personality disorders, dissociative disorders and psychoses usually require a year or more to *reach* enough *stability* to be able to engage in Stage Two work. A trauma survivor may have grown up in an unhealthy, troubled or dysfunctional family. Many survivors may still be in a similar unhealthy environment, whether at home, in one or more relationships, or at work.

How long does the Stage Two recovery process typically take? For a history of trauma that has become entrenched, which most are, it can take years to heal enough to find lasting peace. For some it may take less time. There is no requirement or judgment on the amount of time it takes for a person to recover. It takes as long as it takes. My 28 years of experience in leading trauma-specific therapy groups has been that the members continually find relief when *working* or even when simply *listening* to others' work. In *A Gift to Myself*, I include numerous guidelines and experiential exercises to help facilitate Stage Two work, with a section at the end on how to access when it may be time to stop therapy.

It is helpful to make a personal recovery plan, a point I have emphasized throughout my prior books. Making such a recovery plan gives us lots of advantages as we heal, one of which is to discover the usefulness of naming things accurately (see the Chapter, "Naming Things Accurately," in *A Gift to Myself* for details). For example, instead of "depression," if appropriate, consider calling it grieving from major losses and/or childhood trauma. And instead of saying "I deserved it," consider calling it abuse or trauma. These kinds of reframes can be effective as we heal. Doing so is important because what we deal with in therapy is often actually grieving, or stuck grief, and not "depression" or

176

another "mental disorder." "Depression" and "mental disorder" involves *Stage Zero* and *Stage One thinking*, and reframing depression as stuck grief—that is, needing to grieve but being somehow blocked from doing it—would be more accurate Stage Two thinking and understanding. As a therapist, coming from that understanding, we can see the need to help people identify and accurately name exactly what they are grieving from or about, thereby aiding them in their healing in a healthy way.

What about a person who can't do more therapy because of managed care restrictions, budget constraints, low income and so on? We do the best with what we have. People who are motivated to heal can be creative. That's one reason *I wrote my books*—that is, *for my patients*, so they could save time and money by learning how to do the healing themselves, although with the help of safe others, including some therapists. Often, people go from one therapist to another, like people do with attempted intimate relationships. Some fit. Others don't. They learn as much as they can with one teacher or guide and then go on to the next.

STAGE THREE

Stage Three recovery involves spirituality and its incorporation into daily life. Folding this strong recovery aid into our everyday flow is an ongoing and lifelong process. Stage Three is learning to realize spirituality. It is expanding the same question, "Who am I?" from Stage Two work, since that is a central question there, too. In Stage Three, the person is continuing to work on "Who am I?" in a deeper way. But now we also expand that question, "Who am I?" to the next interesting one: "What am I doing here?" and then "Where am I going?" Actually, Stage Three encompasses the whole process, from Stage Zero onward. Everything we do is spiritual, and by spiritual I am not talking about religion. I'm talking about relationships and experiences with self, others, and the Universe or God/Goddess/All-That-Is. Spirituality is about making meaning that may involve different levels of our life. [163,177,178]

Spirituality is a powerful tool. If the recovering person or their therapist does not understand spirituality, then one of the best places to learn about it is in most any Twelve Step fellowship group, no matter what the focus. Many people confuse spirituality with religion. While religions are kinds of "brand names," spirituality is the generic umbrella that embraces and transcends all religions. Psychological health is one of its goals. The healthier we are, the easier we can stay directly and authentically connected to ourselves and our Higher Power. [164,165]

Having a spiritual connection to God, i.e., a sense of connection to a Higher Power, may be an association or aid for suicide prevention. For example, psychiatrist C. Bruce Greyson and Barbara Whitfield conducted research on 20 patients who attempted suicide and were admitted to the psychiatric unit at the University of Connecticut Hospital. Those who had near-death experiences, in which they had a direct and powerful positive experience with a Higher Power, usually did not attempt suicide again. [163] They commonly said that they now had a sense of "cosmic unity." Other studies have replicated these results. Suicide attempters who did not have a near-death experience, but who were given books to read about it, developed some of the same positive aftereffects and attitudes. Working a Twelve Step program may lead us in the same direction, as numerous authors have described and countless people have experienced directly.

Many to most clinicians do not address the patient's nutritional intake, their exercise activity, or their spiritual life–all of which can affect our emotional and behavioral experiences and symptoms, and our quality of life. Most do not know that adequate dental/oral health for those labeled as being "mentally ill" is important, although it is. ³ This and other seemingly unimportant aspects of a healthy lifestyle will strengthen our long-term recovery, as reflected above on page 111 to 113 and in the next section.

DIAGNOSIS AND THE RECOVERY STAGES

The *DSM* and similar diagnostic schemes, codebooks and categories are useful mostly in Stages Zero and One. They can have some usefulness in Stage Two recovery, such as in the case of alerting clinicians when people may have a personality disorder or another one to which they may need to pay special attention. In all of these stages, *DSM* diagnoses are also useful for insurance reimbursement purposes, since the insurance industry requires a codified diagnosis before it will pay for health care. Beyond these considerations, I believe that the *DSM* diagnostic categories are not very useful. They are useless in Stage Three recovery work and, except for the above situations, in most of Stage Two. Even so, throughout this book, I refer to these diagnostic labels for purposes of accuracy in describing the strong associations that these forms of "mental illness" have with people with a history of childhood and subsequent trauma. I do this to point out how close mental illness was and is to repeated childhood and later trauma.

I'm not alone in these observations and opinions, as six colleagues' examples (Kutchins & Kirk, [87] Caplan, [193] Ross, [132] Bremner, [28] Middleton [200] and Zur [185]) have described *clear problems* and *deficiencies* with the formulation and usefulness of the *DSM*.

Regarding its relationship to childhood trauma, Bremner said:

"This hypothesis of a common neurological deficit [among trauma survivors] could explain why there is such overlap among many disorders, and why clinicians are frustrated with the current diagnostic schema. The past half-century of psychiatry has been

179

largely absorbed with an attempt to force clinicians to accept a "splitters" approach to psychiatric diagnosis which has led to finer and finer splitting of psychiatric diagnoses with successive versions of the DSM. An important foundation of this evolution of the psychiatric diagnosis is the *absence* of any theoretical *foundation* for diagnosis. This was largely a reaction to the previous era, in which psychoanalysis dominated psychiatric diagnosis and imbued a heavily dogmatic and theoretical foundation for it. However, cutting ourselves off from any theoretical foundations has had its price. It has led us into our currently *absurd position* of trying to justify why *multiple* psychiatric *diagnoses*—all spawned from the back of the *DSM* like the heads of the Hydra that sprouted after the single head called 'anxiety neurosis' was lopped off by the so-called biological psychiatrists—are actually distinct entities when all of the evidence points to the contrary. This situation has led us close to a grassroots revolution, in which the clinicians who actually see the patients are ready to assassinate the number crunchers who developed this idiotic scheme and are forcing the clinicians to comply with it in the name of 'consistency of diagnosis' or 'research protocol.' In fact, these clinicians started ignoring the *DSM* years ago. However, if queried, they will spout the dogma like Protestants challenged by Catholic inquisitors in Spain during the fourteenth century. The fact is that it is time for us all to wake up and realize the truth—that these disorders are not truly distinct, that they have a common basis in neurology [i.e., trauma effects], and that we need to take a more enlightened approach to their evaluation and treatment." [28] [my italics]

This is a telling observation, one that many trauma-aware clinicians have often made. Bremner concludes,

"Of course, the most relevant rationale to strengthen ourselves in terms of diagnosis is so that we can appropriately treat patients with trauma-related psychiatric disorders. If we can properly diagnose trauma patients [as trauma survivors], we can apply the correct treatments for these disorders. We are starting to learn more about treatments for trauma-related disorders, and the good news is that some treatments we have learned about in the past few years show considerable promise for disorders such as PTSD."

This leads us into the mental disorders other than depression that are commonly found to be variations among the effects of trauma. Indeed, some have suggested that if the *DSM* were to be rewritten with the truth about trauma effects more realistically in mind and told, it would become much smaller and most of it would consist of subcategories of a common diagnosis such as "post-trauma syndrome, manifested by fill-in-the-blank". [28,87,132,185,193] To bridge that conceptual gap, in my two books *The Truth About Depression* and *The Truth About Mental Illness,* I provide an even firmer base from which to understand the multiple guises of the effects of repeated trauma.

AVOID PSYCHIATRIC DRUGS

Referring to the 5th recovery action above: **No psychiatric drugs,** I have described nearly all psychiatric drugs as being non-specific in their actions. A major reason why most commonly prescribed psychiatric drugs are non-specific in their actions and don't work well is because they do not hit the target at which they are aimed, i.e., at one or more presumed mental illness(es). Instead, nearly all of these drugs tend to detrimentally effect many if not most of our organs, functions, and useful human faculties outside of or in addition to the target symptom or symptoms. In that sense they have been called "shotgun" drugs. It is as though a marksman is shooting at a target to hit the bulls eye (the symptom or "mental illness" alone) with a single bullet, but instead hits most everything outside the target (i.e., the drug's toxic effects, which

181

BigPharma and the other Bigs disguise by calling them "side effects"). In this sense a psych drug's shotgun blast at times may hit *parts* of the target, but it also hits almost everything else in the area in and around the area in which the target sits, including the trees, the ground and any animals or humans who may be in the background (Figure 14.1). These surrounding areas are analogous to many to most of the body's organs, including the brain, nervous system and the mind and its crucial functioning capacities.

Figure 14.1

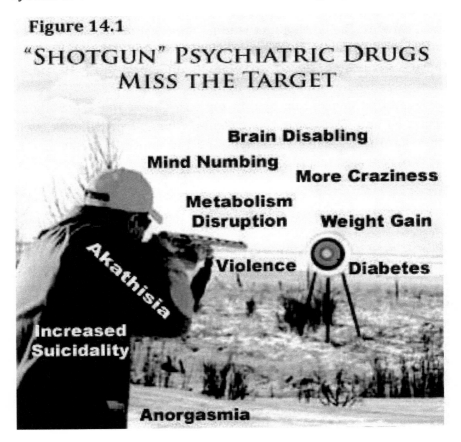

"SHOTGUN" PSYCHIATRIC DRUGS MISS THE TARGET

Psychiatric drugs neither treat nor cure any "mental illness." What they "treat" are simply psychiatric symptoms—but at a price—by disabling the brain, mind, emotions and our decision-making abilities, and thereby *inducing* an *abnormal brain state*. I summarize this situation in Table A.11 on drug action *theory* versus their *actual effects* in the Appendix on page 223.

Research and clinical psychiatrist Joanna Moncrieff says that most psychiatrists advocate biological psychiatry's theory which focuses on clusters of psychiatric symptoms as though they represent distinct psychiatric disorders (middle column of Table A.11 on page 223) which she calls a *disease-centered* theory for psychiatric drug action. But she and an increasing number of others, including e.g., Peter Breggin, others and I, disagree with that *disease-centered* theory. Instead we see nearly all psychiatric drug's actions as what Moncrieff calls *drug*-centered, as summarized in the right-hand column of the table. Many psychiatrists claim that using these drugs is analogous to using the drug insulin for diabetes, attempting to suggest that psychiatric drugs are real and disease-specific biological chemicals such as insulin and that psychiatric diseases/disorders are real biological entities as diabetes is. They implicate to their patient that they will therefore need whatever psychiatric drug(s) they have prescribed—a not so subtle suggestion that they will need the drug(s) for life no matter how toxic they may be. Could this be a kind of authoritative indoctrination that manipulates countless patients daily across the world into believing that they actually need the drug(s)?

By contrast, Moncrieff's *drug-centered* view is analogous to using alcohol for social phobia or social anxiety. Here Breggin's quote from his classic 2008 book *Brain-disabling Treatments in Psychiatry* bears repeating: "People commonly use alcohol, marijuana and other non-prescription drugs to dull their feelings. Usually they do not fool themselves into believing they are somehow improving the function of their minds and brains. Yet when people take psychiatric drugs, they almost always do so without realizing that the drugs 'work' by disrupting brain function, that the drugs cause withdrawal effects, and that they frequently result in dangerous and destructive mental reactions and behaviors." Most of us know that alcohol's effect is as a dose-dependent anesthetic agent that will kill if we drink enough acutely and over time. But too few know that the same principle applies in varying degrees to nearly all psychiatric drugs, including if taken at low doses over time. See Grace Jackson, Joanna Moncrieff and Peter Breggin's work for details, plus my article "Psychiatric drugs as agents of trauma" in *The International Journal of Risk and Safety in Medicine* (2010). [25,80,81,173,174,179]

CONCLUSION

In this chapter I summarize the essentials of the process of healing and recovery from the painful effects of trauma —the effects that conventional clinicians today routinely misdiagnose and mistreat as though they were one kind or another of "mental illness." I provide the details for each of the 10 recovery principles and the 5 actions of this healing process in several of my other books: *Healing the Child Within, A Gift to Myself, Boundaries and Relationships* and *My Recovery*: A Personal Plan for Healing. Other of my books that may help are: *Memory and Abuse, The Truth about Depression, The Truth about Mental Illness*, and for an in depth description of core issues in recovery in my new book *Wisdom to Know the Difference.*

After having read this chapter, consider referring back to pages 19 to 22 to review and correlate that information in the text and flow chart as Figure 2.1.

In the next chapter I discuss one of the most important aspects of recovery and day-to-day life: the importance of getting a good quality and amount of sleep every night.

15   The Importance of Good Sleep

To live a healthy life, most of us need to spend a third of our day and thus our life in normal good sleep. A normal night's sleep consists of *at least* three **periods** of five sleep **stages** that include cycles of delta, alpha, theta, and REM (Rapid Eye Movement) sleep, each period/cycle usually lasting about 90 to 110 minutes (1.5 to nearly 2 hours.) It is normal to wake up periodically during the night between these cycles and of course, it is normal to get up to empty our bladder once or twice nightly. Dreaming tells us that we are asleep (when in REM sleep) or early in a sleep cycle (called "hypnogogic" dreaming). Whether they are normal or scary (nightmares), dreams serve us to **process** and **release uncompleted emotional conflicts from the day before**. We don't have to remember or always analyze our dreams because as we dream we process our previous day's emotional conflicts in each dream. [66]

If we so sleep and dream, the next day we will usually be rested, awake and alert. If we don't, we often feel tired, un-rested and unable to face the day as productively. Good sleep also **balances** and **strengthens** our immune, nervous, endocrine, and other body systems. Sleep recharges and re-energizes our psychological, emotional, spiritual, and physical batteries.

SLEEP AMONG TRAUMA SURVIVORS

Others and I have shown how trauma survivors are commonly misdiagnosed as being "mentally ill" and then mistreated.[173,174] Most trauma survivors don't sleep well. We commonly have a restless night and wake up feeling un-rested and fatigued, and too often are unable to concentrate on our daily tasks. We may thereby feel a related loss of peace and joy in our life. **Lack of good sleep** commonly aggravates our quality of life the next day and **over time may simulate many of the symptoms of "mental illness."**

Difficulty sleeping is a hallmark of PTSD. [99,102] Among the *diagnostic criteria* of PTSD regarding disturbed sleep are:

• **Difficulty falling or staying asleep,**
• **Recurrent distressing dreams** of a traumatic event, and
• **Acting or feeling as if a traumatic event were recurring** ... **even** when that occurs **upon awakening during the night**. Other diagnostic criteria can be involved when the sleeper awakens and can't go back to sleep from
• **Over-stimulation due to bothersome fears or other worries** that are part of their distress during their waking life. [135] I summarize and expand these observations in Table 15.1.

Table 15.1 Sleep problems in PTSD

(compiled from Singareddy & Balon 2002) [148]

Problem	*Description*
Insomnia	• Difficulty falling asleep • Difficulty staying asleep • Feel un-rested in morning
Nightmares	• Trauma related nightmares • Other nightmares
Worrying & other	• Negative imagination • Startle/fear awakenings without dreams • Restless legs/ Sleep-related breathing disorders • Thrashing movements • REM sleep behavior disorder • Drug effects

Repeated trauma leads to PTSD, which results in poor sleep. Inadequate sleep then leads to difficulty functioning the next day, and if repeated for days, weeks, months, or even years can aggravate or worsen the PTSD, and depending on the individual, **often** manifests as what *appears* **to be "mental illness."** The insomnia and mental illness is then usually mistreated with toxic and addicting **psychiatric drugs**, which in turn **can worsen sleep, mind** and **body**.

SLEEP HELPS MOOD, MEMORY AND CONCENTRATION

Have you ever done an "all nighter" to study for an exam, only to find that during the test you could barely remember what you had studied? Good sleep helps us organize memories, solidify learning, and improve our concentration. Where we actively dream in REM sleep, our body-mind regulates our mood. Poor sleep can make us irritable, emotional, and make bad decisions. Sleep deprivation also affects motor skills, enough to be similar to drunk driving if we are seriously sleep deprived. Driver fatigue causes over 100,000 accidents and 1500 deaths each year. [194]

STAGES AND CYCLES

Our sleep is regulated by an internal body clock that is sensitive to light, time of day and other cues for sleep and awakening. Sleep cycles throughout the night, moving back and forth between deep restorative sleep and more alert stages and dreaming. As the night progresses, we spend more time dreaming and in lighter sleep REM sleep is when we do our most active dreaming. Non-REM (NREM) sleep consists of four stages of deeper and deeper sleep (Figure 15.1). Each sleep stage is important for good sleep, but deep sleep and REM sleep are especially vital.

Figure 15.1 Sleep cycle example

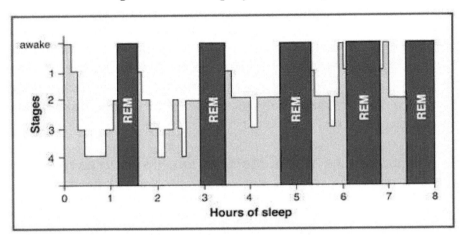

DEEP SLEEP

Each sleep stage helps us. Deep sleep may be the most vital. The strongest effects of sleep deprivation are from inadequate deep sleep—the first stage that the brain attempts to recover when we are sleep deprived. What disrupts deep sleep? Some examples: If we are caring for someone around the clock, whether it is a small infant or an elderly relative with a serious illness, we might need to attend to them suddenly in the middle of the night. Loud noise outside or inside the home might wake us. If we work a night shift, sleeping during the day may be difficult, due to light and excess noise during the day. Substances like alcohol and nicotine also disrupt deep sleep.

To maximize our deep sleep we can make our sleep environment as comfortable, quiet and dark as possible. If we are being awakened as a caregiver to another or others, we can get some more time of uninterrupted sleep, especially if we have had disruptive nights.

REM SLEEP

REM (dream) sleep is essential to our minds for processing and consolidating our emotions, memories and stress. It is also vital to learning, stimulating learning and developing new skills. Most of our dreaming occurs during REM sleep, although it can happen during other sleep stages as well. There are different theories as to why we dream. Freud, Jung and their colleagues thought that dreams process our long-held unconscious conflicts. Today, many believe that it is the brain's way of processing random fragments of information received during the day. [66] If REM sleep is disrupted one night, our body will go through more REM the next to catch up on this sleep stage. Much of dreaming is still a mystery. [88]

GETTING MORE REM SLEEP

Studies have shown that better REM sleep helps boost our mood during the next day. To get more REM sleep we can try to sleep a little more in the morning. As our sleep cycles through the night, it starts with longer periods of deep sleep. By morning REM sleep is longer. Try sleeping an extra hour and see if your mood improves. Improving overall sleep will also increase our REM sleep. If our body is deprived of deep sleep, it will try to make that up first - at the expense of REM sleep.

Many things can cause or aggravate insomnia and interfere with good sleep. I list some of the more common of these in Table 15.3. One of the most common causes of insomnia is PTSD, which itself is characterized by several factors that interrupt sleep (Table 15.1 above).

As described throughout this book and elsewhere, [173] many to most mental disorders have PTSD underlying them and can be understood as being variations of the many faces of PTSD.

Figure 15.2 Brain waves during sleep stages

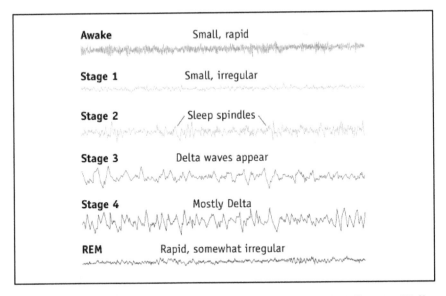

From Saisan J, de Benedictis T, Barston S, Segal R 2009 Sleeping Well
helpguide.org/life/sleeping.htm

Another common cause of insomnia is the use of **psychiatric drugs** that due to their direct toxicity or through drug withdrawal **may interfere** with good sleep (Table 15.3). While the makers of these drugs may claim that they help people sleep, and some may do so for a time—such as is claimed with the tricyclic antidepressant trazodone—many of them actually often *interfere* with healthy sleep. Ambien and similar "sleep aids" (see Table 9.3 on page 106), actually interfere with REM sleep.

Restless leg syndrome (RLS) causes insomnia by its repetitive painful paresthisias (worse-than-ordinary tickling-like sensations) in the lower legs throughout the night. It usually affects one leg at a time more than the other and often later in the night shifts to the other leg. Each episode lasts for several seconds and re-occurs

Charles L. Whitfield, M.D.

about every 28 seconds, often temporarily relieved by moving the effected leg, but still preventing going deeper into good sleep.

Table 15.2 Sleep stage characteristics [88]

Sleep Stage	Brain waves Frequency & Amplitude	Description
0 Waking state	Alpha fast, low	"Awake" most of day
1 Drowsiness	Theta Begin to be slower & deeper	Lasts 5-10 minutes. Eyes and muscles move slowly, easily awakened.
2 Light sleep	Become even slower & deeper	Eye movements stop, heart rate & body temp decreases
3 & 4 Deep	Delta waves Slowest & deepest	Difficult to awaken; if awakened, do not adjust immediately & often feel groggy & disoriented for several minutes. Allows brain to go on short break to restore the energy we expend when awake.. Brain blood flow decreases, & redirects towards the muscles, restoring physical energy. Immune functions increase
5 REM Dreaming	REM Faster & less deep	70 to 90 minutes into sleep cycle, usually three to five REM episodes per night. Associated with processing emotions, retaining memories & relieving stress. rapid, irregular and shallow breathing, heart rate & blood pressure rises, males erections, females clitoral enlargement.

RLS can be relieved by taking chelated magnesium and manganese supplements, sometimes by acetaminophen (Tylenol) and usually by getting up and walking around. Another cause of insomnia is **sleep-related breathing disorders**, such as sleep apnea and the like.

Table 15.3 Common interferences with sleep

Interferences	Causes & Description
PTSD	**Insomnia common** to **usual.** As described in text. [148]
Drug effects **Antidepressants**	These block certain sleep stages, from deep sleep to REM sleep *Toxicity:* **Severe anxiety, agitation, insomnia, overstimulation. sleep deprivation, hangover.** Akathisia (severe, painful stimulation & inner restlessness); mania
Antipsychotics	*Withdrawal:* **insomnia**, depression, **anxiety, agitation, restlessness, panic**, labile mood, crying spells, easy irritability, hostility, aggression, impulsive behavior, akathisia, **vivid or bizarre dreams**, mania, hypomania; **restless legs**, hypomania to mania, headache; abdominal pain
Benzodiazepines; other sedatives; sleeping pills & alcohol	*Toxicity:* confusion, blurred vision, **anxiety, agitation,** hallucinations, altered mental status, impaired thinking, confusion, delirium, disinhibition, including extreme agitation, psychosis, paranoia *Withdrawal:* **Anxiety, panic, insomnia, restlessness, agitation,** emotional lability, irritability, muscle: tension, spasms, cramps; **insomnia,** "brain zaps," clouded consciousness, confusion, "psychosis," disorientation, derealization, paranoia, hallucinations, delusions, "depression," hyperactivity
Anti-convulsants, aka "mood stabilizers"	**Toxic effects**, including **withdrawal** insomnia, headache, nausea

Table 14.3 Common interferences with sleep ... *continued*

Stimulants [25]	***Toxicity:* Insomnia**, headaches, nausea, **anxiety**, irritability, abdominal pain, psychosis, mania, hyperactivity, depression, withdrawn, permanent neurological tics/spasms, incl. Tourette's syndrome, Palpitations, tachycardia ***Withdrawal:*** Insomnia, anxiety, agitation, nausea, abdominal cramps, paranoia, psychotic symptoms, hallucinations, delirium
Opiates **Chronic pain**	***Toxicity:*** Dysphoria ***Withdrawal*: anxiety, irritability, insomnia, restless legs**, physical pain. Numerous causes, often treated with opiates
"Mental illness" – various	PTSD commonly underlies most of them. Commonly misdiagnosed & mistreated
Restless Legs Syndrome	Common. Esp. in opiate withdrawal, ADP & Antipsychotic WD, magnesium & manganese deficiency
Sleep-related Breathing Disorders	Can be severely disruptive to good sleep.
Light & Noise	We sleep best in total darkness & silence. Leaving any lights or noises on such as TV or radio interferes with our ability to get good sleep.

We sleep best in total darkness and silence. Leaving any lights or noises on in our bedroom such as the television or radio usually interferes with our ability to get good sleep. I have seen many

---

[25] Include Ritalin, Adderral, and the like, plus cocaine, caffeine, nicotine, psychedelics, corticosteroids & some broncho-dilators used in asthma.

trauma survivors who said the only way they could sleep was with having a light and TV or radio on.

Table 14.4 Sleep interference from drugs

Sleep Phase	Drugs Interfering
Decrease REM sleep	Antidepressants (tricyclics & SSRI/SNRIs), lithium, benzodiazepines, phenobarbital, diphenhydramine (Benadryl), opiates, β-blockers, dopamine agonists, [26]
Increase waking after sleep onset	Opiates, prednisone, clonidine, diuretics, β-blockers, stimulants
Increase stage 2 sleep	Antidepressants (tricyclic), phenobarbital
Non-specific interference	Antipsychotics, stimulants, incl. psychedelics, caffeine & nicotine. Many "sleeping pills" incl. eszopiclone (Lunesta) & Zolpidem (Ambien)

Some sleeping pills such as eszopiclone (Lunesta), Zolpidem (Ambien) and benzodiazepine sedatives may help temporarily, but too often result in chemical dependence, which then makes insomnia worse due to withdrawal. When the person stops taking them they usually experience bothersome withdrawal symptoms, including an often worsening insomnia.

Psychiatric drugs, including sleeping pills, thus interfere with our sleep in these several ways and can block our dreaming significantly. Tracy says that from an increasing dream deprivation over time (remember that dreams have a bizarre, surreal and often psychotic content) our thus distressed nervous system can trigger or try to dream for us during the day, which can manifest as

---

[26] α-methyldopa (Aldomet) increases REM sleep

hallucinations or other psychotic symptoms or signs, leading to another misdiagnosis and mistreatment. [199]

AN APPROACH TO GOOD SLEEP

In my medical practice I have found a generic approach to attaining better sleep by using sleep hygiene and selected nutritional and physiological supplements, as described below.

1) Take "Melatonin Plus," 3 mg, or regular **melatonin** 3 mg and 100 mg **L-theanine** one hour before bedtime. You can substitute for the melatonin with a low dose, one teaspoon **tart cherry concentrate** in a half-glass water, 20 minutes before bedtime.

• ***Keep another such half-glass ready*** *at your bedside to drink if you wake up in the middle of the night and can't go back to sleep.* [Can order tart cherry concentrate from Obstbaum.com and elsewhere online; keep it in your freezer.] And/or can take an extra 5-HTP (see next).

• If the above doesn't work, or if you have more serious insomnia, add number 2 below.

2) In addition to the above, also take 100 mg of **5 HTP**, similar to tryptophan, an hour before bedtime.

• If that doesn't work, continue by increasing the dose of either melatonin and/or 5 H Tryptophan by one extra dose.

• If that doesn't work for you, add number 3 below.

3) Add to all of the above 500 mg of **GABA** an hour before bedtime.

• If that doesn't work, add number 4 below.

4) Add Passion flower 300 mg or more an hour before bedtime. [178]

• If that doesn't work, add number 5 below.

5) Add to all of the above Tylenol PM or Advil PM (have Benadryl added – caution hangover & withdrawal insomnia).

If these don't work, you might try adding any of the supplements from Table 15.5 below *one at a time*.

These above supplements and summarized in Table 15.5 are psychoactive in that they make us sleepy or sedated. Simulating the body's normal physiology, they are biologically active in our body, especially in our brain and nervous system. Many and possibly most of these supplement drugs appear to act on a receptor site or they appear to stimulate other sites in the flow of our body's metabolism. They are relatively more addiction free and are specific for calming or sedating —as compared with other psychoactive drugs such as antidepressants, antipsychotics, benzodiazepines and the like, which are highly addicting and generally toxic to our nervous system and body, and over time often make it harder for us to sleep well.

Avoid caffeine intake, in the form of coffee, tea, sodas or chocolate (including cocoa) or energy shots or drinks at any time. If you have to have a morning dose of caffeine, limit it to one dose only before noon.

If you are taking any other stimulant drugs, including antidepressants, these may disrupt your sleep. If any concerns, avoid alcohol and other drugs—legal or not legal.

Exercise during the day (but not in the evening) will usually help us sleep better.

Bedroom should be as dark and quiet as possible, no TV, no blinking lights from electronic components.

Table 15.5 Supplements and drugs to help sleep

(most taken an hour before bedtime)

Supplement	Dose	Comments
Melatonin	1 to 3 mg or more	Body's own natural sleep aid; decreases with age
5 HTP	100 to 300 mg	Amino acid anti-anxiety & sedative agent
l-theanine	100 mg or more	Amino acid anti-anxiety agent; may potentiate melatonin effect; may help some with OCD
GABA	100 mg or more	Amino acid anti-anxiety agent & sleep aid
Passion flower extract	200 mg or more	Herbal anti-anxiety & sedative agent
Tart cherry concentrate	1 tsp in ½ glass H_2O	Anti-anxiety effect in 15 minutes, lasts about 4 hrs. Keep mixed at bedside for later if can't go back to sleep
Valerian root/extract	2-3 gm /2-300mg	Mild to moderate sedative properties
Clonidine	0.1 to 0.3 mg *prescription only*	Anti-hypertensive drug with sedative effects. Helps lessen opiate withdrawal.
diphenhydramine	25-50 mg	Trade name Benadryl; hangover, withdrawal & addiction possible.
Magnesium (Mg) &/or **manganese**	As directed on bottle	May help some people sleep. Chelated Mg or Mn works better.

*Can order all inexpensively from Vitacost.com 800-381-0759

Another help is learning to relax and self-sooth while waiting for sleep. Worrying can be replaced by simple prayer. Say to yourself or a safe other person what is bothering you and then "turn it over" to God. The only rule here is that once you have asked for help in prayer—you don't need to ask again. Ask for help with your worry and "turn it over."

BODY CHECK AND POSITIVE THINKING

You can also do a "body check" every so often while waiting for sleep to come. Start at your toes and slowly go up your body sensing tight muscles or feeling any stress. Ask for it to release. Once you experience the stress releasing you can do this repeatedly when you become aware of it. In the beginning this will happen several times. Watch your breathing while you are doing this. Breathe into your belly. Shallow breathing (just the chest moves) contributes to stress. Belly breathing helps blow off stress. Take three breaths into your belly and then relax your breathing.

Now watch your thoughts. Instead of going into story lines that pop up spontaneously, try telling yourself that now you are totally relaxed and drifting off to sleep. Repeat how comfortable your body is and believe it. Keep focused on these simple exercises to prevent your attention from wandering off again.

Post-traumatic stress disorder (PTSD) may be the most common cause of insomnia and is often aggravated by sleep deprivation. They fuel each other in a cycle that can be broken by doing the above and getting well rested. Of course the effects of PTSD combined with sleep deprivation commonly simulate or masquerade as "mental illness." When we get good sleep, these effects improve, and for many they go away.

APPENDIX I

TABLE A.1 ANTIDEPRESSANT & ANTIPSYCHOTIC TOXICITY

ADPs/SSRIs	Antipsychotics
Psychiatric/Psychological	
Depression or **worsening of depression, suicidal thoughts, gestures,** or **completed,** esp. in **children** & **teens.** Suicidal overdose. **Sedation,** may be marked Severe **anxiety, agitation, overstimulation. Insomnia, sleep deprivation, hangover. Akathisia** (severe, painful stimulation & inner restlessness). Parkinson's disease, **tardive dyskinesia, involuntary movement disorders, dystonia,** seizures, **brain damage,** Obsessions and compulsions; may motivate **violence** toward oneself or others. **Temper tantrums, screaming, aggression** Both also have → **Psych drug stress-trauma syndrome. Withdrawal,** mild to **severe**	
Mania, ± **psychotic features,** e.g., hallucinations, delusions, psychosis, out-of-control behavior, including sexual acting out, road rage, spending sprees ["bipolar"] and shoplifting. **Violence** and other criminal acts. Elevated mood, euphoric, or irritable. Hypomania. "Serotonin" syndrome (Restlessness, hallucinations, nausea, diarrhea, headache, shivering, diaphoresis, confusion, coma)	**Mental, emotional & psychic blunting, numbing, slowed thinking & talking, disinterest, indifference, lack of spontaneity & motivation, lethargy, apathy,** social withdrawal, **poor concentration** (chemical lobotomy), **dysphoria.Unalert.** Iatrogenic (treatment-caused) learned **helplessness. Learning difficulty** (alert: children & teens), **Decreased working memory** (blackouts). ↑ **Appetite, compulsive eating** (see *Somatic*)

All **Boldface** items = more common

→ **Toxicity manifestations** *continued on the next page*

Table A.1 Antidepressant & Antipsychotic Toxicity
... continued

ADPs/SSRIs	Antipsychotics
Neurologic Stroke, bleeding, frontal lobe syndrome (apathy, indifference, loss of initiative &/or disinhibition), myoclonus; restless legs; loss of balance, **falling, broken bones**	↓ **brain volume**; torticollis, **oculogyric crisis**, opisthotonus; In short are chemical straight-jackets Other: Low physical activity, substance abuse, unprotected sexual activity
Somatic **Weight gain, sometimes severe**, with blood sugar ↕ imbalance, **diabetes**; pancreatitis; liver damage; heart problems; urinary incontinence. **Loss of libido, erectile dysfunction, anorgasmia**. Male breast enlargement ± breast cancer. Neonatal toxicity, birth defects; neonatal/newborn drug withdrawal	Heart arrhythmias, sudden death, **earlier than normal death**, respiratory depression, orthostatic hypotension, may be severe, esp. in overdose. **Weight gain, sometimes severe**, with blood sugar ↕ imbalance, **diabetes** Neuroleptic malignant syndrome * Amenorrhea, galactorrhea, hyperprolactinemia, sexual dysfunction, breast cancer, osteoporosis. Hyperthermia, urinary retention, intestinal ileus, mydriasis, toxic psychosis, dry mouth, hot, dry flushed skin.

The **withdrawal** of monoamine oxidase inhibitors (**MAOIs**) can result in severe anxiety, agitation, pressured speech, sleeplessness or drowsiness, hallucinations, delirium, myoclonic jerks, and paranoid psychosis. MAOI withdrawal phenomena resemble the symptoms produced by the discontinuation of chronically administered stimulants, [such as amphetamines].[27]

---

[27] Acta Psychiatrica Scandinavica 78 (1) , 1–7 1988

TABLE A.2 ANTIDEPRESSANT & ANTIPSYCHOTIC *WITHDRAWAL* TOXICITY

Antidepressants (ADPs)	Antipsychotics
Psychiatric/Psychological **Difficulty focusing, confusion, forgetfulness,** incoherence, **derealization, depression, anxiety, panic, labile mood,** crying spells, **easy irritability, agitation, restlessness,** hostility, aggression, **impulsive behavior, akathisia, suicidality,** drowsiness, **insomnia,** vivid or bizarre dreams, mania, **hypomania**	
Feelings of unreality, depersonalization - sense of unreality and **loss of self**	Auditory or visual **hallucinations, paranoid delusions,** grandiosity, elation, delirium & other psychotic symptoms
Neurologic Dizziness, vertigo, tremors, **paresthesias** (including electric shock-like tingling or pain), restless legs, lowered libido, movement disorders (**akathisia,** Parkinsonism), **tardive dyskinesia** (repetitive, disfiguring movements of face, head, tongue, neck, limbs, trunk) or worsening of it, tremor, dystonias, difficulty walking, behavioral activation from **hypomania** to mania, headache, amnesia	
Somatic **Nausea,** vomiting, anorexia, diarrhea, **fatigue, lethargy,** sweating, **myalgias (muscle aches)** or ridigity, rhinorrhea, weakness	
Sweating, muscle spasms, malaise, hot or cold flashes, shaking chills, palpitations, heart arrhythmias	Fever, stomach pain All **Boldface** items = **common**

Diagnostic Steps for Psychiatric Drug Withdrawal

1) History or suspicion of patient's **stopping** psychiatric drug(s)

2) Patient's **symptoms and signs match** withdrawal symptoms and signs above

3) If in doubt, **therapeutic trial** of low to moderate dose of suspected drug

4) Know that chances of success in withdrawal are good if patient has a good **support system** to help them withdraw and not interfere with the process

5) Awareness of **external pressures** to go back on drug (esp. family & other clinicians/authorities)

6) Careful **monitoring** of clinical course

* Depression, anxiety, psychosis, or other "mental illness" symptoms and signs (see all above & other tables) may be a **feature of drug withdrawal** rather than the re-emergence of an underlying illness.

* Reactivation of underlying PTSD may mimic drug withdrawal, "mental illness," and/or be a *part of both*.

— See Table A 3 on next page

TABLE A.3 ANTIDEPRESSANT WD v. DEPRESSION v. PTSD ACTIVATION

Observation	Antidepressant Withdrawal	"Depression"	PTSD Activation
Stop ADP or reduce dose	Within 2-3 days 35–78% patients	Uncommon in first week	Within 2-3 days Common
Onset	Abrupt, sudden	Gradual	Abrupt, sudden
How long on ADP	Weeks to months	No set time	
Symptoms	See withdrawal Sx table	Conventional depression Sx	PTSD Sx almost identical (see TaD)
Response to ADP (same drug) dose	Sx improved by 2 to 24 hours	Slow, over several days to weeks	Depends on data in previous 2 columns
MisDx'd as Depr. or another disorder	Can lead to misTx with more/different drug(s) → DSTS*	Initial ADP effect may burn out	May be the correct diagnosis
Complications	• Physical Sx Dx → waste $, risk, misDx Sx as med problem • DSTS*	May lessen a positive response to drug	Aggravates PTSD symptoms
PTSD history	Common if looked for carefully		By definition
Cautions	• Don't stop any psych drug suddenly • High suspicion of symptoms as drug WD • Initially R/O PTSD; be mindful of DSTS		· Avoid most psych drugs; Use non-drug recovery aids

*DSTS = Drug Stress Trauma Syndrome; Sx = Symptom(s);
Dx = Diagnosis; Tx = Treatment; R/O = Rule Out; WD = Withdrawal;
Depr = Depression; TaD = *The Truth about Depression*

TABLE A.4 STIMULANTS & BENZODIAZEPINES TOXICITY

Stimulants: Ritalin, Adderall, etc	Benzodiazepines: Valium, Xanax, Klonopin, etc
Toxic Effects **Sleep disorders**, headaches, **decreased appetite**, nausea, anxiety, **irritability,** abdominal pain. Psychosis, mania, chemical dependence, inattention, hyperactivity, depression, withdrawn, **overfocusing, robotic behavior,** permanent neurological tics/spasms, incl.Tourette's syndrome, **growth retardation** via growth hormone disruption, brain trophy (shrinkage), other permanent brain damage. Palpitations, tachycardia, and increases in diastolic and systolic blood pressure. **Suppression of spontaneity, creativity, and healthy independence.** Substance use disorders in adolescence. *Legal:* Many commit a **felony,** end up in **mental institutions** or **prisons** by 18 YO. The "ADHD" label may limit career choices incl. military, law enforcement, etc	*Toxic Effects* *Acute:* **Dizzines, confusion, drowsiness, blurred vision, unresponsiveness, anxiety, agitation, nystagmus,** hallucinations, slurred speech ataxia, coma, hypotonia, weakness, altered mental status, impaired thinking, confusion, delirium, *disinhibition*, including extreme agitation, psychosis, paranoia, and depression, sometimes with violence toward self or others; **amnesia/blackouts,** paradoxical agitation, respiratory depression, hypotension *Chronic:* **Emotional blunting or numbing,** decreased memory & concentration, forgetfulness, **habituation, chemical dependence,** impairment of visual-spatial ability and attention span, everyday brain dysfunction, brain atrophy → **Withdrawal manifestations** *shown on the next page*

Charles L. Whitfield, M.D.

Stimulants: Ritalin, Adderall, etc	Benzodiazepines: Valium, Xanax, Klonopin, etc
Withdrawal Effects **Depression**, exhaustion, **suicidality, lethargy, apathy, difficulty focusing, insomnia**, drowsiness, **anxiety**, agitation, nausea, abdominal cramps, paranoia, psychotic symptoms, pressured speech, hallucinations, delirium	**Withdrawal Effects**[28] **Fear, anxiety**, panic, **insomnia**, apprehension, **restlessness, agitation, emotional lability, irritability, muscle: tension, spasms, cramps; insomnia, "brain zaps"*** clouded consciousness, **confusion**, "psychosis," disorientation, derealization, depersonalization, **paranoia**, hallucinations, delusions, **"depression,"** suicidality, hyperactivity, **decreased memory & concentration**, i.e., "ADHD" symptoms, anorexia, **paresthesias** (sometimes bizarre), sensitivity to light, sound, touch, pain, feeling of motion, tinnitus, metallic taste, fever, seizures, **drug craving**
Any or all of above → leading to **misdiagnosis** of other "mental disorders," including "dual disorders") & thus mistreatment with **other toxic** psych drugs → from which **more withdrawal** symptoms will be likely, leading to even more **misdiagnosis** of other "mental disorders" → viscious cycle. We can call this resulting repeated & associated physical & emotional pain the **Drug Stress Trauma Syndrom**e	

[28] On withdrawing from benzos or antidepressants, "brain zaps" are brief but repeated electric shock-like sensations in the head, or extending elsewhere in the body. Sometimes accompanied by disorientation, tinnitus, vertigo and lightheadedness.

TABLE A.5 LITHIUM & "MOOD STABILIZER" TOXICITY
(aka Anti Epilepsy Drugs)

Lithium	Anti Epilepsy Drugs aka "Mood Stabilizers"
Toxicity - these Sx mean *High* Li toxicity **Brain & Nervous System - Sedation,** confusion, **disorientation, lethargy, mental slowness, social isolation,** *impaired* : **intellect, learning, memory, creativity** **Anxiety, tremor, ataxia** (loss of balance), **myoclonus, muscle rigidity, muscle twitching, hyperreflexia,** tinnitus, blurred vision, Parkinson's disease, headache, seizures, psychosis, coma, death **GI tract -** nausea, vomiting, **diarrhea** **Kidneys – Mild damage** to kidney failure, may be permanent; polydipsia **Other –** Hypothyroidism, **weight gain,** hyperparathyroidism, heart damage, pain, aplastic anemia, dermatitis, ulcers, alopecia *Withdrawal* (discontinuation syndrome) **CNS stimulation, anxiety, fear,** headache, suicidality, hypomania, manic behavior, depression, **dysphoria,** insomnia. *Including -* **Eventual improved sleep,** mental & physical **functioning,** & **quality of life** for most who can handle the emotional pain & be patient in a full recovery program. **Close follow-up therapy is crucial.**	**Valproate** (Depakote, etc) – **Weight gain, dyspepsia,** endocrine, liver, serious blood toxicity, fetus & brain damage, fatigue, peripheral edema, dizziness, drowsiness, hair loss, headaches, nausea, **sedation,** tremors **Carbamazepine** (Tegretol) -- **Drowsiness, ataxia, upset stomach,** serious blood, skin & fetus toxicity, liver disease, heart problems **Gabapentin** (Neurontin) -- **Dizziness, drowsiness,** peripheral edema, liver, kidney toxicity; **mood swings,** suicidality, hyperactivity, hostility, **difficulty focusing** **Topiramate** (Topamax) – **Mood** *problems*: **anxiety, sedation, fatigue, dizziness; problems with:** focus/attention, aggressive behavior [all "ADHD" like], **coordination, vision, memory & speech,** sensory distortion, anorexia, weight loss, metabolic acidosis; fetus & brain damage, **anemia, psychosis, suicide attempt;** drug interactions (common among all AEDs)

Lithium	Anti Epilepsy Drugs aka "Mood Stabilizers"
See Withdrawal symptoms *and advantages to tapering and stopping at bottom left of the above table section.* *Do not taper or stop any psychiatric drug without expert medical supervision.*	**Lamotrigine** (Lamictal) -- **Memory loss**, word-finding difficulty, taste change, **URIs**, emotional blunting, **paresthesias, lethargy**; kidney stones, impaired motor skills, transient or permanent vision loss, fatigue, **osteoporosis, headache, dizziness, insomnia**, anxiety; depression, **nausea, diarrhea**, constipation, retarded growth **Olanzapine** – Brain atrophy, other antipsychotic toxicity (see attached) **Phenytoin** (Dilantin) -- Ataxia (loss of balance) at overdose, skin, gum problems - rare *Withdrawal* (discontinuation syndrome) for *all above* (though minimal for phenytoin): **CNS stimulation, anxiety, fear, seizures, other; improved health is common**

All **Boldface** items **=** more common

TABLE A.6 OPIATES & NICOTINE TOXICITY

Opiate Drugs (painkillers): heroin to oxycontin	Nicotine (cigarettes, cigars, chew, snuff, patch) - the most commonly used psych drug (along with alcohol)
Toxic Effects **Acute: High dose** "Overdose" Sedation, inability to function, respiratory depression, cyanosis, shock, pinpoint pupils, decreased urine formation, hypothermia, pulmonary edema, death. **Lower dose** Many using low to moderate doses, report early on increased **energy**, courage, **confidence**, & **euphoria**. But these "positive" effects gradually - usually over days to weeks to months wear off (drug tolerance) - leaving the user with painful withdrawal (see below) which causes craving for relief by more opiates. Other, perhaps "lucky" early opiate users experience discomfort and dysphoria and stop before bothersome withdrawal sets in. **Chronic:** Constipation, sedation, inactivity, (alternating with constant and repeated drug seeking) irritability, emotional outbursts, hostility, aggressive behavior, violence, emotional roller coaster effects, financial difficulties, stealing for money.	**Toxic Effects** **Acute:** Marked central nervous stimulation, tremors, nausea, vomiting, vasoconstriction throughout body, abdominal pain, diarrhea, cold sweat, headache, dizziness, disturbed hearing and vision, mental confusion, weakness, low blood pressure, fast and week pulse, collapse, death. **Chronic:** Early death, chronic obstructive pulmonary disease (COPD), inability or difficulty to feel feelings, especially fear, guilt, shame and anger. Underneath these are often hurt, sadness and emptiness. **Highly toxic** to most organ systems: stroke, sudden death, heart attack, asthma, chronic bronchitis, emphysema, **Cancer** of the lung, mouth, throat, espophagus, stomach, pancreas, uterus, cervix, kidney, ureter, bladder; OBGyn toxicity: ectopic pregnancy, spontaneous abortion, infertility, impaired fetal growth and development;, repeated nicotine withdrawal, drug seeking behavior, empty promises to quit. **Toxic to bystanders**

Table A.6   Opiates & Nicotine   *...continued*

Opiate Drugs (painkillers): heroin to oxycontin	**Nicotine** (cigarettes, cigars, chew, snuff, patch) - the most commonly used psych drug (along with alcohol)
Withdrawal Effects Craving for opiates, **restlessness**, incl. **restless legs, anxiety, irritability, insomnia**, dysphoric mood, increased sensitivity to pain, nausea, vomiting, **diarrhea, muscle aches**, stomach **cramps, back pain, sweating**, piloerection ("gooseflesh"), dilated pupils, impulsivity, **difficulty concentrating**, yawning, tearing, fever, high blood pressure; protracted withdrawal and body aches and pains over days to 2 weeks.	*Withdrawal Effects* **Easy irritability**, anger, **fear & anxiety, difficulty concentrating**, low energy, coughing, **drug seeking** behavior, weight gain, **low tolerance for emotional pain.** One of the most difficult of all psychoactive drugs to stop. **Gradually improved quality of life**

SPELLBINDING

One major effect of the commonly used psych drugs (antipsychotics, anti depressants, benzodiazepines and often lithium and the anticonvulsants, often erroneously called "mood stabilizers") is what psychiatrist and author Peter Breggin calls "spellbinding." Spellbinding means that the drugs blunt the person's awareness or appreciation of their drug-influenced mental dysfunction. It is a kind of chemical dissociation or separation from reality. Too often this drug effect makes the person misperceive that they are improved or even doing better than ever, when in fact, they are no better and often doing worse than they did before they took the drug.

Breggin observed that "This brain-disabling principle of psychiatric treatment is not a speculation. It is a solid scientific theory based on hundreds of evidence-based reports, clinical experience, and commo sense observations." Others and I agree with his observations and statements. [25,109,186]

He continues: "In the extreme, medication spellbinding drives individuals into bizarre, out-of-character destructive actions, including suicide and violence. Medication spellbinding is an aspect of the brain-disabling principle that explains why so many individuals [continue to] take drugs of all kinds, from antidepressants to alcohol, when they are causing them great harm and even destroying their lives."

Spellbinding is a built-in effect of most psychoactive and psychiatric drugs that reinforces the coercive power of each of the kinds of forced drugging in Chapter 10. I summarize these effects, including how they are related to dependence and withdrawal, in the table on the next page.

TABLE A.7 THE SPELLBINDING EFFECT OF PSYCHOACTIVE DRUGS & ITS RELATION TO DRUG WITHDRAWAL (EXPANDED FROM BREGGIN 2006, 8)

Drug Type	*Effects Summary*	*Dependence/ Withdrawal*
Antidepressants	• Stimulation (common; mania in extreme) &/or sedation (less common) • Mental & emotional dulling, esp. LT* • Violence, suicide, over-stimulation	Many to most can't stop due to WD** Depends on drug
"Mood Stabilizers" aka anticonvulsants; lithium	Sedating, dulling &/or stupefying; depression, suicide, over-stimulation;	Many can't stop due to WD
Antipsychotics aka neuroleptics	• Severe frontal lobe inhibition, negative trance. • Less able to think & act for self • "Chemical lobotomy," zombie-like, robotic, dementia, severe agitation (akathisia), withdrawal psychosis	Many to most can't stop due to WD
Benzodiazepines	• Sedation to euphoria, mental & emotional dulling, depression, cognitive impairment; • Decreased ST memory*** • Disinhibition of conscience & morality in alc & benzos; psychosis (esp cannabis)	
Alcohol		Common among alcoholics
Cannabis		WD occurs for daily users

Table A.7 The spellbinding effects of psychoactive drugs & its relation to drug withdrawal ...continued

Drug Type	Effects Summary	Dependence/ Withdrawal
Stimulants (Amphetamines to Ritalin to cocaine to nicotine)	Increased energy, limited alertness, agitation, mental & emotional dulling LT, mania, "OCD." apathy psychosis, over-focusing, depression	Many to most can't stop due to WD
Opiates aka "Narcotics"	Sedation to euphoria Increased energy (antidepressant) for some	Hard to stop if use LT
Phencyclidine (PCP, "angel dust")	Severe negative global brain effects, psychosis	Rare to use LT
All psychoactive drugs (legal & illegal)	• Stimulation to sedation; • Mental & emotional dulling &/or stupefying • Impaired judgment • Cognitive impairment • Fail to sense their impairment • False sense of well-being • Lobotomy effect	Many to most can't stop LT without WD by *slow dose* decrease (over months). Clinical supervision recommended for withdrawal

* LT = Long Term; ** WD = bothersome to serious withdrawal from drug; *** ST = Short Term

Depending on length of exposure and dose, many to most people in withdrawal from psych drugs can**not** usually stop on their own. The difficulty is mostly due to the facts that:

1) they and their clinician do not know how to recognize drug withdrawal,

2) the emotional and physical pain of the drug withdrawal are often more painful than the original symptoms such that the *only* way for them to get emotional and physical *pain relief* is to *continue* taking the *drug*.

Along with other factors, spellbinding starts and maintains the chemical dependence that often develops to most psychoactive drugs. The drug's dulling, dampening, and blunting of our mind and feelings—and the withdrawal (usually undiagnosed and untreated)—commonly assure that the person will continue to use the drug(s). Most clinicians misdiagnose actual drug withdrawal as though it is instead a relapse of the original symptoms (which they commonly misinterpret as being a re-emergence of the original disease or disorder – or as a new one), thus maintaining the drug use and any resulting toxicity.

Appendix II for PTSD

PTSD DIAGNOSTIC CRITERIA LIMITATIONS: We can define a traumatic experience in many different ways. What is a trauma to one person may not be traumatic to another. Before recovery, a person might define a trauma differently than that person might do after being in recovery for a while. And during recovery our understanding of what a trauma is often changes. In 1980, the original *DSM-III* committee defined a trauma as a "recognizable stressor that would evoke symptoms of significant distress in almost everyone." Seven years later (in a revision, as *DSM-III-R*), they narrowed it down to any event that was "outside the range of usual human experience and that would be markedly distressing to almost anyone". Their major purpose for doing so may have been to distinguish unusual stress, with which most people are unprepared to deal, from everyday stress. Unfortunately, in their most recent definition in the 1994 *DSM-IV* they have focused mostly on the person's physical integrity wherein they react with intense fear, a definition which others and I view as being clinically limiting and inappropriate (see item A in Table 5.2 on page 47).

For example, in the *DSM-III-R* definition (the second one cited above), how easily can we agree on the word *usual*? And how can we determine what "markedly distressing to almost anyone" means? Davidson and others have written about the importance of the subjective perception and appraisal in response to a traumatic event. Two people may respond differently to the same event.

With this more accurate understanding, we can begin to examine the "specific details that need to be understood about each traumatic experience, including the *characteristics* of the *event* itself and the *perceptions, feelings,* and *meanings* for the victim." [173] I and many clinicians who assist trauma survivors prefer to focus more on items B, C, D, E, and especially F from the diagnostic criteria for PTSD (Table 6.2 on page 55). Item F says that "the disturbance causes clinically significant distress or impairment in social, occupational, or *other important areas of functioning*" [my emphasis].

Because others and I have seen countless people who have dissociative amnesia and are not able to remember and name the full *DSM-IV* Category A description that focuses mostly on the person's physical integrity wherein they react with intense fear, we have described it as a PTSD sub-variant (Chapter 5 on page 55).

In Review of Table 5.3 Variants of PTSD [179] from page 55

PTSD Variant	Characteristics and Description
PTSD [179] **Sub-variant**	Little, unclear or no memory of Category A trauma experiences or history. May fulfill less *DSM* diagnostic criteria than required for classical PTSD, yet patient usually has one or more trauma spectrum disorders and other trauma effects.

Charles L. Whitfield, M.D.

TABLE A. 8   MARKETING MYTHS & FACTS ABOUT PSYCHIATRIC DRUGS

Expanded from Breggin 2008a&b, Moncrieff 2008, & Goodman 2007

Myth (Falsehood)	Fact
Mental illness is due to abnormal brain chemistry	There is no definitive or convincing evidence or proof for this claim. See Table A.9 for 18 example statements by authorities.
Psychiatric disorders are diseases like diabetes	False and misleading. There is no laboratory or other objective test or data to back up this claim.
The drugs don't harm the brain permanently	Commonly cause numerous brain, nervous system, and other body defects, from cell damage or cell death to tardive dyskinesia (bothersome tremors and movement problems)
In small doses drugs are relatively harmless	Many reports of causing numerous psychiatric symptoms and problems, including violent behavior, on few or low doses (Breggin 2008 a&b)
The drugs are needed to prevent suicide & violence	No convincing evidence. Actually often *cause* suicide and violence
The drug only unmasked your underlying mental disorder	Through the drug's toxic effects, including withdrawal, the drugs actually *cause* psychiatric symptoms which are commonly misdiagnosed as being mental disorders.
You will need to take them for life	There are no "for life" or even long-term studies available. Most drug studies and trials last from 4 to 6 weeks only.
Your psychiatrist is a brain expert	Most know and recite Big Pharma's pseudoscientific claims about the brain and mind.
Your doctor knows what's best for you	Extensive examples of misdiagnosis and mistreatment for "mental illness" refute this myth
TV/magazine drug ads are truthful and helpful	They are simply marketing and sales devices with much false information

215

TABLE A.9 18 QUOTES ON SEROTONIN & ANTIDEPRESSANT DRUGS

Quotation	Source
"Although it is often stated with great confidence that depressed people have a serotonin or norepinephrine deficiency, the **evidence** actually **contradicts** these claims[49]."	Neuroscience Professor **Elliot Valenstein PhD**, in *Blaming the Brain* (1998), which reviews the claims and actual evidence for the serotonin hypothesis.
"Given the ubiquity of a neurotransmitter such as serotonin and the multiplicity of its functions, it is **almost as meaningless to implicate it in depression as it is to implicate blood**[11]."	**Science writer John Horgan**, in his critical examination of modern neuroscience, *The Undiscovered Mind* (1999).
"A serotonin deficiency for depression has **not** been **found** [50]."	**Psychiatrist Joseph Glenmullen**, clinical instructor of psychiatry at Harvard Medical School, in *Prozac Backlash* (2000).
"So far, there is **no** clear and convincing evidence that monoamine deficiency accounts for depression; that is, there is **no "real" monoamine deficit** [43]."	**Psychiatrist Stephen M. Stahl**, in a textbook used to teach medical students about psychiatric medications, *Essential Psychopharmacology* (2000).
"Some have argued that depression may be due to a deficiency of NE [norepinephrine] or 5-HT [serotonin] because the enhancement of **noradrenergic or serotonergic ...transmission** improves the symptoms of depression. However, this is	**Psychiatrists Pedro Delgado** and **Francisco Moreno**, in "Role of Norepinephrine in Depression", published in the *Journal of Clinical Psychiatry* in 2000. **He calls it an Invalid analogy example**

Charles L. Whitfield, M.D.

akin to saying that because a rash on one's arm improves with the use of a steroid cream, the rash must be due to a steroid deficiency[51]."	
"...I wrote that Prozac was no more, and perhaps less, effective in treating major depression than prior medications.... I argued that the **theories** of brain functioning that led to the development of Prozac **must be wrong** or incomplete[52]."	Brown University **psychiatrist Peter Kramer**, author of *Listening to Prozac*, which is often credited with popularizing SSRIs, in a follow-up clarifying letter to the New York Times in 2002.
"I spent the first several years of my career doing full-time research on brain serotonin metabolism, but I never saw any convincing evidence that any psychiatric disorder, including depression, results from a deficiency of brain serotonin. In fact, **we cannot measure brain serotonin** levels in living human beings so there is **no way to test** this **theory**. Some neuroscientists would question whether the theory is even viable, since the brain does not function in this way, as a hydraulic system[53]."	Stanford **psychiatrist David Burns**, winner of the A.E. Bennett Award given by the Society for Biological Psychiatry for his research on serotonin metabolism, when asked about the scientific status of the serotonin theory in 2003.
"Indeed, **no abnormality of serotonin in depression** has ever been demonstrated." [54].The serotonin theory of depression is **comparable to the masturbatory theory of insanity**. Both have been	**Psychiatrist David Healy**, former secretary of the British Association for Psychopharmacology and historian of the SSRIs, in *Let Them Eat Prozac* (2004).

217

depletion theories, both have survived in spite of the evidence, both contain an implicit message as to what people ought to do. In the case of these myths, the key question is whose interests are being served by a widespread promulgation of such views rather than how do we test this theory."	**Sidebar**: After 15 years of extensive studies, as early as 1984 the NIMH said "Elevations or decrements in the functioning of serotonergic systems per se are not likely to be associated with depression."
"We have hunted for big **simple neurochemical explanations** for psychiatric disorders and have **not found** them [55]."	**Psychiatrist Kenneth Kendler** the co-editor-in-chief of *Psychological Medicine,* in a 2005 review article.
Calls the **chemical imbalance** story a "useful metaphor" but says it is **never** one he **uses** when talking to patients. "I can't get myself to say that."	**Psychiatrist Wayne Goodman** (2005), chair of the psychopharmacologic advisory committee of the US Food and Drug Administration, & U Fla Psychiatry
It is high time that it was stated clearly that the **serotonin** imbalance **theory** of depression is **not supported by the scientific evidence** or by expert opinion. Through misleading publicity the pharmaceutical industry has helped to ensure that most of the general public is unaware of this.	**Psychiatrist Joanna Moncrieff**, Senior Lecturer in Psychiatry at University College, London (2005); widely published author
"…there is **no definitive lesion, laboratory test, or abnormality** in brain tissue that can identify the [mental] illness." p. 44 "The precise causes (etiology) of mental disorders are not known." pp. 49 & 102	**Mental Health: A Report of the Surgeon General** (1999) remains true today (2011)

"Although reliable criteria have been constructed for many psychiatric disorders, **validation of the diagnostic categories** as specific entities has **not** been **established**." p. 43 " Most of these [genetic studies] examine candidate **genes** in the **serotonergic pathways**, and have **not** found convincing **evidence** of an association." p. 51	**Hales & Yudofsky** *Textbook of Clinical Psychiatry* 3rd edition (1999)
"In the areas of **pathophysiology and etiology**, psychiatry has more **uncharted territory** than the rest of medicine...Much of the current investigative research in psychiatry is directed toward identifying the pathophysiology and etiology of major mental illnesses, but this goal has been achieved for only a few disorders (Alzheimer's disease, multi-infarct dementia, Huntington's disease, and substance-induced syndromes such as amphetamine-related psychosis or Wernicke-Korsakoff syndrome)."...chapter on schizophrenia: p 23	**Andreasen and Black** *IntroductoryTextbook of Psychiatry* (2001)
"[There are **no**] **biological markers for mental disorders**..." "[There is] **no diagnostic laboratory test** capable of confirming the presence of a mental disorder" "...Brain **science has not**	**American Psychiatric Association** Letter from the APA to a group of clinicians & researchers who challenged their claims of the biological causation model of psychiatry, 26 Sept 2003 On a similar note, a year later, the

advanced to the point where [we] can **point to** readily discernible pathologic lesions or genetic abnormalities that [are] reliable or predictive **biomarkers** of a given mental disorder or mental disorders as a group." "[There **may be**] 'triggering' by certain adverse **environmental influences**. Here, 'environment' **may refer to traumatic events**...."	same group of clinicians & researchers challenged **Pfizer** drug co. to give any **peer-reviewed published evidence** that proved their claim that "Zoloft helps correct the chemical imbalance in the brain of people with depression, PTSD, panic disorder, & OCD." Pfizer was **unable** to **provide** any evidence. (Scientific Panel, MindFreedom Support Coalition International – MindFreedom.org April, 2005)
The truth about mental illness is that it is not as advertised. It is not what some special interest groups tell us. It is not what drug companies and some mental health groups may claim. It is **not simply a group of genetically transmitted disorders of brain chemistry**. It does not reliably respond to psychoactive drugs. And these drugs are not their only available recovery aid.	**Charles L. Whitfield MD** *The Truth about Depression* 2003 & *The Truth about Mental Illness*: Choices for Healing. Health Communications, Deerfield Beach, FL, 2004
"The impact of the **widespread promotion** of the **serotonin hypothesis** should not be underestimated. **Antidepressant advertisements** are ubiquitous in American media, and there is emerging evidence that these advertisements have the **potential to confound the doctor–patient relationship**. ... These advertisements present a seductive concept, and the fact that patients are	**Lacasse JR, Leo J** (2005) Serotonin and Depression: A Disconnect between the Advertisements and the Scientific Literature. **PLoS Med 2(12): e392** [Referance numbers in brackets in left column are for this excellenr article]

now presenting with a self-described **"chemical imbalance"** [46] shows that the DTCA [direct-to-consumer advertising] is having its **intended effect**: the medical marketplace is being shaped in a way that is **advantageous to the pharmaceutical companies**. ...The **incongruence** between the scientific literature and the claims made in FDA-regulated SSRI advertisements is **remarkable**, and possibly unparalleled."	There are many others who have made similar statements to those throughout the left-hand column of this table, including research, forensic and clinical psychiatrists Peter Breggin, Grace Jackson, and others, including some authors writing in the 2009 edition of the state-of-the-art Kaplan and Saddok's 2 Vol. Set *Comprehensive Textbook of Psychiatry*
Summary **From 10 mainstream psychiatrists & the APA, 2 psychiatry texts, 5 scientific observers, & 1 highest US Govt medical source (the *Surgeon General*)**	*Conclusion* - **None of these sources is able to provide any firm evidence for the existence of a biologic or genetic cause for any common psychiatric illness, including the serotonin/norepinephrine neurotransmitter theories. There is no readily available, reliable biologically-based laboratory test for any of them.** **In fact, they affirm the *absence* of evidence for these theories, in spite of the fact that most in psychiatry routinely claim the opposite.**

TABLE A.10 LEGAL EVIDENCE FOR PSYCHIATRIC DRUG TOXICITY
– examples found

Drug/Yearly Sales	Toxicity	Number of Suits/Avg. Amounts Awarded/Total
Paxil 2010 (paroxetine) by Glaxo 11.7 B 9 yrs	Birth defects	>900/1.2M per family/>1 B
	Suicides -Caused	150/ 1.25 per family / 187 M
	-Attempted	300/ 300k per case/ 9 M
	Addiction	3,200/50k per case/ 16 M *
Seroquel ** (quetiapine) AstraZeneca 4.9 B 2009	Diabetes	26,000 / trials pending / 656 M early-on Tentatively settled nearly 4,000 summer 2010
	Suicide	*See also Elliott below*
Zyprexa ** (olanzapine) Eli Lilly 4.2 B in 2006	Diabetes	1,800/ /500 M 28,500/ 27-90k per case /1.2 B 1,200 suits still pending
Neurontin (gabapentin) Pfizer	Suicide , many other toxic effects	>1,000 / trials pending / Unknown early Classic case of dishonest marketing allowed by FDA (see page 218 & 242 of ref 174)

* >4,500 total suits lost. Also Violence: e.g., 6.4 M to survivors where man killed multiple family members & suicide. Same problems are found among all other SSRI and similar antidepressant drugs.
** Illegal marketing suits and convictions/settlements.

Countless lawsuits are filed worldwide and esp. in USA for all sorts of damages to patients and their families due to psychiatric drugs, yet unaware clinicians continue to prescribe them to their patients who like sheep continue to take them as though it was the best remedy for their problems. Lawyers have a system to recruit such clients for which they make from 30 to 50% of each successful suit's awards.
Lawyer website examples: Potential injuries from **antidepressant** side effects include: Suicide attempts, Antidepressant birth defects when taken by pregnant women, Serotonin Syndrome when combined with migraine medication, Increased risk of fractures and bone loss among older adults.
www.youhavealawyer.com/side-effects/antidepressants-paxil-prosac-oloft.html
Call our antidepressant lawyers now at www.1800theeagle.com/topics/Anti-Depressants.html **Antipsychotics** may be included in their search.

TABLE A.11 PSYCHIATRIC DRUG ACTION: THEORY V. ACTUAL EFFECTS*

Characteristic	*Biological* psychiatry theory (disease-centered)	*Actual* drug effect (drug-centered)
Abnormal brain state *theory*	Genetically transmitted brain chemistry defect	No evidence for either part of this theory. (Trauma *can* alter brain)
Drug action on an abnormal brain state	Helps correct the claimed abnormal brain state	***Drug creates*** an abnormal, detrimental brain state
Therapeutic effects are due to	Drug action on presumed disease pathology (abnormal brain state)	Drug-induced abnormal brain state on mental, emotional, behavior problems
Target	**Disease/disorder:** Goal to reduce symptoms by acting on the claimed biological problem that produces them	**Symptoms:** Goal to suppress or overlay symptoms by the abnormal drug-induced state.
Drug effects on Patients v. volunteers	Differ, affect patients, not volunteers	Do not differ
Drug research results	Effect on "disease" & its symptoms	General drug effects
Specific vs. non-specific effects of drug action	Disease specific theory: e.g., "Antidepressant, Antipsychotic, Anti-manic, Mood stabilizer, Anxiolytic" Believe hit the bulls-eye (the "disorder")	Non-specific, "shotgun" effects (miss the bulls-eye but hit all target rings & everything in surrounding area, including innocent bystanders)
Example of analogy	**Attempted:** Insulin for diabetes	**Actual:** Alcohol for social phobia or social anxiety
Best & worst results	"Curative" at best, Palliative (lessens symptoms) or ineffective at worst	Temporarily palliative at best, brain/body & life damaging at worse (common)

*Compiled & expanded from Moncrieff & Cohen 2005; Moncrieff 2008; Breggin 2008a&b; Whitfield 2003,4

IATROGENIC DISABILITY—A DISTURBING TREND

Do psychiatric drugs taken long-term make someone better or worse? Do they increase the likelihood of functioning well long-term, or do they increase the likelihood that a person will end up on disability? *

This is an expansion of my page 139 referral to a dramatic and disturbing trend in the number of people now on disability for "mental illness" over the past 20-plus years. In 2010 Whitaker wrote that "The number of disabled mentally ill has risen dramatically since 1955, and during the past two decades, a period when the prescribing of psychiatric medications has exploded, the number of adults and children disabled by mental illness has risen at a mind-boggling rate. Thus we arrive at an obvious question... Could our drug-based paradigm of care, in some unforeseen way, be fueling this modern-day plague?" [162] (see Figure below)

The Disabled Mentally Ill in the Prozac Era
SSI and SSDI Recipients Under Age 65 Disabled by Mental Illness, 1987–2007

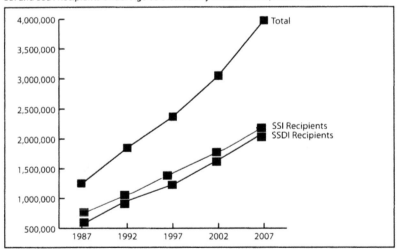

One in every six SSDI recipients also receives an SSI payment; thus the total number of recipients is less than the sum of the SSI and SSDI numbers. Source: Social Security Administration reports, 1987–2007.

To support the Bigs' claims that this "epidemic" is real "mental illness," Whitaker says that "The history must reveal why there has been a dramatic increase in the number of disabled mentally ill, it must explain why disabling affective disorders are so much more common now than they were fifty years ago, and it must explain why so many children are being laid low by serious mental illness today." [162] But it does not. It falls way short of the inter-related facts that: 1) Most of these people are made chronically ill ("disabled") by our current dysfunctional mental health system that misdiagnoses and mistreats them with toxic drugs that make them worse instead of better (see e.g., Drug Stress Trauma Syndrome on page 67); 2) Many to most will have an underlying PTSD &/or active addictions due to repeated childhood and later trauma and which the drugs neither cure nor effectively help; and 3) Enablers from the state and federal government, clinicians, lawyers, and many family members support this debilitating problem. This is a mental health system-induced disability.

A solution is two-fold: 1) Vigilance and taking responsibility for addressing the above 3 facts by each involved person and their clinician, and 2) A creative and effective refocusing by the helping professions onto the areas that I address in this book. Most of the Bigs won't do or allow that, with the only chance for waking up being among academic and professional groups. For that to happen an entire paradigm shift would likely be required. To understand this whole situation takes a good degree of clinical sophistication and an open mind with an ability to "think outside the box."

*Can someone with a mild disorder have a bad reaction to an initial psych drug, which puts them onto a path that can lead to long-term disability? For example, someone with mild depression may have a manic reaction to an antidepressant, and then is misdiagnosed with bipolar disorder and put on several toxic drugs. How often does that happen? Could that be an iatrogenic [physician-caused illness] pathway that is helping to fuel this increase in the disability rates?

FIGURE A.1 SYMPTOM SCORES AMONG CSA SURVIVORS
(broken lines) Compared to Control Sample (bottom, solid line) (from Elliott & Briere 1995, by permission)

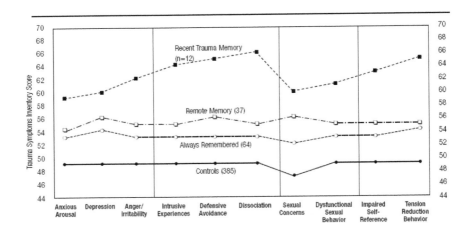

References

1. Abramson J (2005) *Overdo\$ed America:* the broken promise of American medicine. Harper Perennial, New York, NY

2 Abramson J (2006) *Money Talks*: Profits Before Patient Safety with: Bob Goodman ,Alex Sugerman-Brozan, Jeanne Lenzer, Scott Schultz ,Jerome Hoffman http://www.moneytalksthemovie.com/experts.html

3 Arnaiz A, Zumárraga M, Díez-Altuna I, Uriarte JJ, Moro J, Pérez-Ansorena MA. (2010) Oral health and the symptoms of schizophrenia. Psychiatry Res. Nov 3. [Epub ahead of print]

4 Anonymous (2006) Adult Children of Alcoholics [Trauma/Dysfunctional Families]. World Service Organization www.adultchildren.org/ New ACA "Big Book"

5 Akhondzadeh S (2001) Passion flower in the treatment of generalized anxiety: a pilot double-blind randomized controlled trial with oxazepam. J Clin Pharm Ther. Oct;26(5):363-7

6 Anda RF, Brown DW, Felitti VJ, Bremner JD, Dube SR, Giles WH (2007) The Relationship of Adverse Childhood Experiences to Rates of Prescribed Psychotropic Medications in Adulthood. American Journal of Preventive Medicine. 32: 389–94

7 Anda RF, Felitti VJ, Walker J, Whitfield CL, Bremner JD, Perry BD, Dube SR, Giles WH (2006) The Enduring Effects of Abuse and Related Adverse Experiences in Childhood: A Convergence of Evidence from Neurobiology and Epidemiology. European Archives of Psychiatry and Clinical Neurosciences. 256: 174–186

8 Angell M (2005) *The Truth About the Drug Companies*: How they deceive us and what to do about it. Random House Trade Paperbacks, NY

9 Angell M: *Drug Companies and Doctors*: A Story of Corruption. @ website in 2010 www.honestmedicine.com/2009/02/drug-companies-doctors-a-story-of-corruption-by-marcia-angell-md.html

10 Aronson JK (ed) (2006) *Meyler's Side Effects of Drugs*: The International Encyclopedia of Adverse Drug Reactions and Interactions (15th Edition) Elsevier Science

11 Baldessarini RJ (1996). Chapters 18 & 19. Drugs and the treatment of psychiatric disorders. (p 399–459). In JG Hardman & LE Limbird (eds.) Goodman and Gilman's *The Pharmacologic Basis of Therapeutics* 9th ed., McGraw Hill, NY

12 Baldessarini RJ, Viguera AC, Tondo L (1999) Discontinuing psychotropic agents. J Psychopharmacol. 13(3):292-3; discussion 299

13 Baldessarini RJ, Viguera AC (1995) Neuroleptic withdrawal in schizophrenic patients. Arch Gen Psychiatry. Mar;52(3):189-92

14 Baillard M (ed) 2003 *Sleep*: Physiology, Investigations and Medicine. Springer, NY

15 Benzodiazepine half life by UK researcher Heather Ashton www.benzo.org.uk/bzequiv.htm Retrieved 2010-11-30

16 Bent S, Padula A, Moore D, Patterson M, Mehling W (2006). Valerian for sleep: a systematic review and meta-analysis. Am J Med 119 (12): 1005–12

17 Boyd S, (2010) *Mental Illness*: Fact of fiction? Equalism Inc, Cornwall, ON www.susanboyd.ca

18 Hadley S, Petry JJ (April 2003). Valerian. Am Fam Physician 67 (8): 1755–8

19 Kripke DF (December 15, 2007). "Who should sponsor sleep disorders pharmaceutical trials?". J Clin Sleep Med 3 (7): 671–3. PMID 18198797

20 Lunesta withdrawal www.blissplan.com/natural-remedies/sleep-treatment/lunesta-withdrawal/

21 Barber C (2008) *Comfortably Numb*: How psychiatry is medicating a nation. Pantheon Books, NY

22 Berlin HA (2007) Antiepileptic drugs for the treatment of post-traumatic stress disorder. Curr Psychiatry Rep. Aug;9(4):291-300

23 Breggin PR (1998) *Talking Back to Ritalin*: What Doctors Aren't Telling You About Stimulants for Children. Common Courage Press

24 Breggin PR, Cohen D (2000) *Your Drug May Be Your Problem*: how and why to stop taking psychiatric drugs. HarperCollins, NY

25 Breggin PR (2008a). *Brain-Disabling Treatments in Psychiatry*: Drugs, electroshock, and the psychopharmacutical complex. 2nd edition Springer Publishing, NY

26 Breggin PR (2008b). *Medication Madness*: A psychiatrist exposes the dangers of mood-altering medications. St Martin's Press. NY

27 Breggin, P. (2013). *Psychiatric Drug Withdrawal*: A Guide for Prescribers, Therapists, Patients and Their Families. New York: Springer Publishing Co.

Charles L. Whitfield, M.D.

28 Bremner JD (2002). *Does stress damage the brain?* Understanding trauma based disorders from a neurological perspective. Norton, NY

29 Bremner JD, Mletzko T, Welter S, Quinn S, Williams C, Brummer M, Siddiq S, Reed L, Heim CM, Nemeroff CB (2005) Effects of phenytoin on memory, cognition and brain structure in post-traumatic stress disorder: a pilot study. J Psychopharmacol. Mar; 19(2):159-65

30 Bremner JD. (2006) The relationship between cognitive and brain changes in posttraumatic stress disorder. Ann N Y Acad Sci. Jul; 1071:80-6.   Phenytoin ref

31 Bremner JD *Before You Take That Pill*: Why the drug industry may be bad for your health. Avery, 2008

32 Bremner, JD Whitfield CL, Anda R, Lanius R, Schmahl C, Vermetten E (In submission) A new look at trauma-related, or trauma spectrum psychiatric disorders

33 Breslau N, Davis GC, Schultz LR (2003).Post-traumatic stress disorder and the incidence of nicotine, alcohol, and other drug disorders in persons who have experienced trauma. Arch Gen Psychiatry 60(3):289–94

34 130. Briere JN (1996). Treatment of adults sexually molested as children: Beyond survival (Rev. 2nd ed.). New York: Springer

35 Brown D, Scheflin A, Whitfield CL (1999): Recovered memories: the current weight of the evidence in science and in the courts. The Journal of Psychiatry and Law 26:5–156, Spring 1999

36 Brown D, Scheflin AW, Hammond C: *Trauma, Memory, Treatment & Law*. WW Norton, NY, 1997

37 Brown D (2001). (Mis) reprensations of the long-term effects of childhood sexual abuse in the courts. Journal of Child Sexual Abuse 9:79–107

38 Brown GW, Harris T (1978). Social Origins of Depression: A study of psychiatric disorder in women. The Free Press/Mac Millan NY

39 Child Welfare League of America Accessed 6 Nov 2010 @ http://www.cwla.org/programs/researchdata/default.htm

40 Children, drugging: www.lawyersandsettlements.com/features/Psychiatric-Drugging-One.htmltarget=_blank

41 *Co-Dependents Anonymous* [CoDA's "Big Book"] www.codependents.org

42 Cosgrove L, Krimsky S, Vijayaraghaven M, Schneider L (2006) Financial ties between DSM-IV, panel members and the pharmaceutical industry. Psychotherapy & Psychosomatics 75:154-160
43 Courtois C, Ford JD, van der Kolk BA, Herman J (2009) *Treating Complex Traumatic Stress Disorders*: An Evidence-Based Guide. Guilford, NY

44 Cutajar MC, Mullen PE, Ogloff JR, Thomas SD, Wells DL, Spataro J. (2010) Psychopathology in a large cohort of sexually abused children followed up to 43 years. Child Abuse Negl. Sep 30. *Example* **of recent report to add to Table 2.1**

45 Cutajar MC, Mullen PE, Ogloff JR, Thomas SD, Wells DL, Spataro J. (2010) Schizophrenia and other psychotic disorders in a cohort of sexually abused children. Arch Gen Psychiatry. 2010 Nov;67(11):1114-9

46 Dart Center for Journalism and Trauma http://dartcenter.org/ **Many journalists don't understand trauma or drug toxicity. This one addresses trauma. Vera Sherav (see below) understands drug toxicity.**

47 Dierks MR, Jordan JK, Sheehan AH. 2007 Prazosin treatment of nightmares related to posttraumatic stress disorder. Ann Pharmacother. Jun;41(6):1013-7

48 Disorders That Disrupt Sleep (Parasomnias) Emedicinehealth

www.emedicinehealth.com/disorders_that_disrupt_sleep_paras
omnias/article_em.htm

49 Drug Facts 2010   www.a1b2c3.com/drugs/gen008.htm
www.benzo.org.uk/bzequiv.htm

50TeenScreenwww.ahrp.org/cms/index.php?searchword=teen
screen&option=com_search&Itemid=5

51 Elliott DM, Briere J (1995). Post-traumatic stress
associated with delayed recall of sexual abuse: A general
population study. Journal of Traumatic Stress 8: 629–647

52 Ensink B (1992). Confusing Realities: A study on child sexual abuse
and psychiatric symptoms. Amsterdam: Vu University Press.

53 308. Epstein JN, Saunders BE, Kilpatrick DG, Resnick HS (1998). PTSD as a
mediator between etiology, and treatment. Journal of Clinical Psychiatry
47:106–10

54 Everett B, Gallop R (2001) *The Link between Childhood Trauma
and Mental Illness*. Sage Publications, London

55 Fabre LE (1990) Buspirone in the management of major
depression: a placebo-controlled comparison. J Clin Psychiatry
51:55-61 suppl

56 Felitti VJ, Anda RF, Nordenberg D, Williamson DF, Spitz AM,
Edwards V, Koss MP, Marks JS (1998). Relationship of childhood
abuse and household dysfunction to many of the leading causes
of death in adults. Amer J Preventive Medicine,14, 24

57 Felitti VJ, Anda RF (2010) Chapter 8. The Relationship of
Adverse Childhood Experiences to Adult Medical Disease,
Psychiatric Disorders, and Sexual Behavior: Implications for
healthcare. in R Lanius & E Vermetten eds. *The Impact of Early
Life Trauma on Health and Disease*:The Hidden Epidemic.
Cambridge U Press

58www.dailytidings.com/apps/pbcs.dll/article?AID=/20100618/N
EWS02/6180314/-1/NEWSMAP
www.ahrp.org/ahrpspeaks/OvermedUSkids0605.php

59 Friedrich WN (1998) Behavioral manifestations of child sexual abuse. Child Abuse & Neglect 22 (6): 523–31

60 Gelman S *Medicating Schizophrenia*: a history. Rutgers U Press, New Brunswick, NJ, 1999

61 Girdano D, Everly G (1979). Controlling stress and tension: A holistic approach. Prentice Hall, NY

62 Glenmullen J (2006) *The Antidepressant Solution*: A step-by-step guide to safely overcoming antidepressant withdrawal, dependence, and "addiction." Free Press, NY

63 Gold SN, Tursich M, Michaels L, Stewart LM, with discussant Whitfield CL. (2010, October). Are the memory wars over? Recent findings and new data on delayed recall. Symposium presented at the International Society for the Study of Trauma and Dissociation 27th Annual Conference, Atlanta, GA.

64 Goodwin J, McCarthy T, Divasto P (1981). Prior incest in mothers of abused children. Child Abuse & Neglect 5:87–96

65 Gottstein JG (2007) Psychiatrists' Failure to Inform: Is there substantial financial exposure? Ethical Human Psychology and Psychiatry, Volume 9, Number 2, 117-125

66 Griffin J, Tyrrell I 2004 *Dreaming Reality*: How dreaming keeps us sane, or can drive us mad. HG Publishing, London
A Modern Classic on dreaming

67 Guntrip H (1973). *Psychoanalytical Theory, Therapy and the Self*. Basic Books/Harper Torch Books, NY

68 Haddad P, Lejoyeux M, Young (1998) A Antidepressant discontinuation reactions. British Medical Journal 316:1105-1106 (11 April)

69 Hall W, Bergman C, McNamara J, Sorensen P(2007) *Harm Reduction Guide to Coming Off Psychiatric Drugs*. The Icarus Project and Freedom Center, NY and Boston

70 Harris G "Leading Psychiatrist Didn't Report Drug Makers' Pay," The New York Times, October 4, 2008.
http://www.nytimes.com/2008/10/04/health/policy/04drug.html
http://www.nytimes.com/2010/10/27/business/27drug.html?_r=1
&ref=gardiner_harris re Paxil

71 Herman JL (1997). *Trauma and Recovery*. Second Edition Basic Books, NY

72 Harper J (2005) *How To Get Off Psychiatric Drugs Safely.* CreateSpace, TheRoadBack.org

73 Healy D, Tranter R (1999) Pharmacological stress diathesis syndromes. Psychopharmacol.;13(3):287-90
74 Healy D, Savage M, Michael P, Harris M, Cattell D, Carter M, McMonagle T, Sohler N, Susser E (2001). Psychiatric service utilisation: 1896 & 1996 compared. Psychological Medicine 31, 779–790

75 Healy D (2004) *Let Them Eat Prozac*: The unhealthy relationship between the pharmaceutical industry and depression. New York University Press

76 Healy D (2008) *Mania*: A short history of bipolar disorder. Johns Hopkins University Press

77 Hollister LE (1999) Pharmacological Stress Diathesis Syndromes: Commentary. J Psychopharmacology 13:293-4

78 Inaba D, Cohen WE (2007) *Uppers, Downers, All Arrounders.* Cns Productions

79 Inman DJ, Silver SM, Doghramji K (1990) Sleep disturbance in PTSD: a comparison with non-PTSD insomnia J Traumatic Stress 3:3

80 Jackson GE *Reconsidering Psychiatric Drugs*. Author House, Bloomington, IN 2005

81 Jackson GE (2009) *Drug-Induced Dementia*: a perfect crime. Author House, Bloomington, IN

82 Joseph J (2003). *The Gene Illusion*. PCCS Books, London

83 Kaplan & Sadock's (2009) *Comprehensive Textbook of Psychiatry*, Vols I & II, Wolters Kluwer/Lippincott Williams & Wilkins, NY.
An egageing mix of excellent real psychiatry and unfortunate drug pushing.

84 Karon B, VandenBos GR (1981) *Psychotherapy of Schizophrenia*: The Treatment of Choice. Jason Aronson

85 Key opinion leaders search (2010) —On Nemeroff www.pharmalot.com/2010/07/nimhs-insel-on-nemeroff-i-regret-my-actions/On others articles.latimes.com/2008/oct/04/science/sci-doctors4

86 Klein-Schwartz W (2002) Abuse and toxicity of methylphenidate. Current Opinion in Pediatrics: Therapeutics and toxicology 14:2 219-2 April

87 Kutchins H, Kirk S (1997). *Making us crazy*: DSM the psychiatric bible and the creation of mental disorders. New York: The Free Press. **See page 179 for comments**

88 Lader M, Cardinali DP, Pandi-Perumal SR 2005 *Sleep and sleep disorders*: a neuropsychopharmacological approach. Springer, NY

89 Laing RD (1965) *The Divided Self:* An Existential Study in Sanity and Madness.Penguin Psychology, London

90 Lamarche LJ, De Koninck J. 2007 Sleep disturbance in adults with posttraumatic stress disorder: a review. J Clin Psychiatry. Aug;68(8):1257-70

91 Lane CJ, Ngan ET, Yatham LN, Ruth TJ, Liddle PF (2004) Immediate effects of risperidone on cerebral activity in healthy subjects: a comparison with subjects with first-episode schizophrenia. J Psychiatry Neurosci. Jan; 29(1):30-7

92 Lanius RA, Vermetten E, Pain C (2010) *The Impact of Early Life Trauma on Health and Disease*: The hidden epidemic. Cambridge University Press

Charles L. Whitfield, M.D.

93 Laplanche J, Pontalis JB (1973). *The Language of Psycho-analysis*. WW Norton, NY

94 Leavitt F (2002). Personal communication. Chicago

95 Legal summary cites 2010 selected: **Paxil** ref:
www.businessweek.com/news/2010-07-20/glaxo-said-to-have-paid-1-billion-over-paxil-suits.html
Seroquel refs: 1) www.businessweek.com/news/2010-02-05/astrazeneca-facing-26-000-lawsuits-over-seroquel-update2-.html 2) www.bloomberg.com/news/2010-07-30/astrazeneca-says-almost-4-000-seroquel-claims-settled-through-mediation.html
Neurontin: www.businessweek.com/news/2010-04-01/pfizer-said-to-settle-neurontin-suicide-lawsuit-for-400-000.html
Zyprexa:query.nytimes.com/gst/fullpage.html?res=9f00e5db1430 f936a35752c0a9619c8b63 Aug 8 2010

96 Lehman J (2010) www.thetotaltransformation.com/ How to set limits with difficult kids. Excellent for unruly kids all ages

97 Lehmann P (2005) *Coming Off Psychiatric Drugs*: successful withdrawal from neuroleptics, antidepressants, lithium, carbamazepine and tranquillizers. Peter Lehmann Publishing, Germany

98 Levine BE (2008) Exposed: Harvard Shrink Gets Rich Labeling Kids Bipolar. AlterNet. Posted June 18; see also
http://www.alternet.org/health/141369 and
http://www.digitaljournal.com/article/276135

99 Levitt AJ, Schaffer A, Lanctot KL, (2009) Chapter 31.12 Buspirone. in Kaplan & Sadock's *Comprehensive Textbook of Psychiatry*, Vol. II, page 3060-5, Wolters Kluwer/Williams & Wilkins (Cite's **buspirone's effectiveness** for treating **PTSD** in articles by Wells et al 1991, Duffy & Malloy 1994, Fichtner & Crayton 1994; Effectiveness in treating **depression** by Fabre 1990, Rickles et al 1990, Robinson et al 1990, Appelberg et al 2001; and 8 references for effectively treating generalized **anxiety** disorder)

100 Liddle PF, Lane CJ, Ngan ET (2000) Immediate effects of risperidone on cortico-striato-thalamic loops and the hippocampus. Br J Psychiatry. Nov;177:402-7

101 Lowinson JH , Ruiz P, Millman RB, Langrod JG (2004) Substance Abuse: A comprehensive textbook, 4th ed. Lippincott Williams & Wilkins, Baltimore

102 Maher MJ, Rego SA, Asnis GM. 2006 Sleep disturbances in patients with post-traumatic stress disorder: epidemiology, impact and approaches to management. CNS Drugs 20(7):567-90

103 Mellman TA, Bustamante V, Fins AI, Pigeon WR, Nolan B. 2002 REM sleep and the early development of posttraumatic stress disorder. Am J Psychiatry Oct;159(10):1696-701

104 Miller A (2008) *The Drama of the Gifted Child*: The Search for the True Self. Basic Books, NY 2008

105 Miller DD 2004 Atypical Antipsychotics: Sleep, Sedation, and Efficacy J Clin Psychiatry 6 [suppl 2]:3–7)

106 Mindfreedom www.mindfreedom.org/ One of the few self-help resources & groups for anyone in the mental health system

107 Mishory A, Winokur M, Bersudsky Y (2003) Prophylactic effect of phenytoin in bipolar disorder: a controlled study. Bipolar Disord. Dec; 5(6):464-7

108 Moynihan R, Cassels A (2006) Selling Sickness: How the world's biggest pharmaceutical companies are turning us all into patients. Nation Books, NY

109 Moncrieff J *The Myth of the Chemical Cure*: A critique of psychiatric drug treatment. Palgrave/MacMillan, UK & NY2008

110 Moncrieff JA 2009 *A Straight Talking Introduction to Psychiatric Drugs*. PCCS Books, Ross-on-Wye, UK

111 Moncrieff J Why is it so difficult to stop psychiatric drug treatment? It may be nothing to do with the original problem. Med Hypotheses. 2006;67(3):517-23. Epub 2006 Apr

112 Morton N, Browne KD (1998). Theory and observation of attachment and its relation to child maltreatment: a review. Child Abuse Negl 1998 Nov; 22 (11):1093–104

113 Najavitz LM, Weiss RD, Shaw SR (1997) The link between substance abuse and posttraumatic stress disorder in women: A research review. Amer. J. Addict. 6: 273-283

114 Najavits LM, Weiss RD, Shaw SR (1999) A clinical profile of women with PTSD and substance dependence. Psychology of Addictive Behaviors 13:98-104

115 Natural News http://www.naturalnews.com/index.html

116 Ngan ET, Lane CJ, Ruth TJ, Liddle PF (2002) Immediate and delayed effects of risperidone on cerebral metabolism in neuroleptic naïve schizophrenic patients: correlations with symptom change. J Neurol Neurosurg Psychiat. Jan;72(1):106-10

117 NIDA National Institute on Drug Abuse 2010 www.drugabuse.gov/infofacts/tobacco.html

118 Noblitt R, Perskin Noblitt P (2008) *Ritual Abuse in the Twenty-First Century*: Psychological, Forensic, Social, and Political Considerations. Robert Reed Publishers

119 Nutt DJ, King LA, Phillips LD (2010) Drug harms in the UK: a multicriteria decision analysis. The Lancet, 376/9752:1558-65, 6 November

120 Oaks DW (2010) Let's Stop Saying "Mental Illness"! http://www.mindfreedom.org/kb/mental-health-abuse/psychiatric-labels/not-mentally-ill

121 Ouimette PC, Kimerling R, Shaw J, Moos RH (2000). Physical and sexual abuse among women and men with substance use disorders. Alcoholism Treatment Quarterly 18, 7–17

122 Ouimette PC, Wolfe J, Chrestman, KR (1996). Characteristics of PTSD-alcohol abuse comorbidity in women. Journal of Substance Abuse 8, 335–346

123 Pandi-Perumal SR ed (2008) *Sleep Disorders*: Diagnosis and Therapeutics. Informa HealthCare, London

124 Pennebaker JW (2000). Telling stories: the health benefits of narrative. Literature and Medecine 19(1):3–18

125 Picken AL, Berry K, Tarrier N, Barrowclough C (2010) Traumatic events, posttraumatic stress disorder, attachment style, and working alliance in a sample of people with psychosis. J Nerv Ment Dis. 2010 Oct;198(10):775-8.

126 Preskorn SH (2003) Relating clinical trials to psychiatric practice: part II: the gap between the usual patient in registration trials and in practice. J Psychiatr Pract. Nov; 9(6):455-61

127 pharmalot.com/2008/10/why-grassley-is-investigating-emorys-nemeroff/

128 Read J, Fink P, Rudegeair T, Felitti V, Whitfield C (2008) Child maltreatment and psychosis: A return to a genuinely integrated bio-psycho-social mode. Clinical Schizophrenia & Related Psychoses. October p. 235-254

129 Rie HE, Rie ED, Stewart S, Ambuel JP (1976) Effects of Ritalin on underachieving children: a replication. Am J Orthopsychiatry. Apr 46(2):313-22; and J Consult Clin Psychol. 1976 Apr;44(2):250-60

130 Ries RK, Miller SC, Fiellin DA, Saitz R (Editors) (2009) *Principles of Addiction Medicine* 4th ed, Lippincott Williams & Wilkins, Baltimore

131 Robinson DS, Rickels K, Feighner J, Fabre LF Jr, Gammans RE, Shrotriya RC, Alms DR, Andary JJ, Messina ME (1990) Clinical effects of the 5-HT1A partial agonists in depression: a composite analysis of buspirone in the treatment of depression. J Clin Psychopharmacol. Jun;10(3 Suppl):67S-76S

132 Ross C, Pam A (eds.) (1995). *Pseudoscience in Biological Psychiatry*: Blaming the body. John Wiley, NY

133 Ross RJ, Ball WA, Dinges DF, Kribbs NB, Morrison AR, Silver SM, Mulvaney FD 1994 Rapid eye movement sleep disturbance in posttraumatic stress disorder. Biol Psychiatry. 1994 Feb 1;35(3):195-202

134 Rothschild B (2000) *The body remembers*: the psychophysiology of trauma and trauma treatment. New York: Norton

135 Saigh PA, Bremner JD (1999). *Posttraumatic Stress Disorder*: a comprehensive text. Allyn & Bacon, NY

136 Samaha AN, Seeman P, Stewart J, Rajabi H, Kapur S (2007)"Breakthrough" Dopamine Supersensitivity during Ongoing Antipsychotic Treatment Leads to Treatment Failure over Time. The Journal of Neuroscience, March 14 (11):2979-2986 —Provides another basis for why these drugs make people worse [179]

137 Scaer RC (2005) *The trauma spectrum*: hidden wounds and human resiliency. New York: Norton

138 Scaer RC (2002) *The Body Bears the Burden*: Trauma, Dissociation, and Disease. Haworth Press, NY

139 Schaler JA (2004) *Szasz Under Fire*: The Psychiatric Abolitionist Faces His Critics. Open Court, Chicago

140 Selye H (1974). *Stress without Distress*. Lippincott, NY

141 Sharav V (2010) Website on BigPharma exploiting vulnerable children and adults: www.ahrp.org

142 Sharav V (2005) America's overmedicated children. Accessed Nov 2010 — Plus see her other many excellent articles and posts
http://www.ahrp.org/ahrpspeaks/OvermedUSkids0605.php

143 Shuster L (1961) Repression and de-repression of synthesis as a possible explanation of some aspects of drug action. Nature 189:314-5

144 Siegel JM. 2003 Why we sleep. Sci American, Nov issue

145 Silverman E (2008) on Key Opinion Leaders, see - www.pharmalot.com/2008/06/senate-targets-stanford-psychiatrist-over-conflicts/   —see also: www.pharmalot.com/

146 Simeon D, Loewenstein R (2009). Dissociative Disorders. in Sadock, Sadock & P. Ruiz (Eds.), *Comprehensive Textbook of Psychiatry* (9th ed, Vol. 1, pp. 1965-2026). Philadelphia: Wolters Kluwer/Lippincott Williams & Wilkens

147 Simos BG (1979). *A Time To Grieve*: Loss as a universal human experience. Family Services Association of America NY

148 Singareddy RK, Balon R. 2002 Sleep in posttraumatic stress disorder. Ann Clin Psychiatry. Sep;14(3):183-90
Sleep stages figure from www.sleepdex.org/stages.htm

149 Smith D, Wesson D (1970s to present) Many talks and papers on upper-downer syndrome re psychoactive drugs. San Francisco and nationally

150 Spiegel D (1990). Hypnosis, dissociation and trauma: hidden and overt observer. In Singer JL (ed.) *Repression and Dissociation*, Univ Chicago Press

151 Spiegel D (1993). Dissociation and trauma. In Spiegel D (ed.) *Dissociative Disorders*: A clinical review. Sidran Press, Lutherville, MD

152 Summit RC (1983). The child sexual abuse accommodation syndrome. Child Abuse & Neglect 7:177–193

153 Szasz T (1984) *The Myth of Mental Illness:* Foundations of a Theory of Personal Conduct (Revised Edition). Harper Perennial

154 Tarrier N (2010) Cognitive behavior therapy for schizophrenia and psychosis: current status and future directions. Clin Schizophr Relat Psychoses. Oct;4(3):176-84

155 Tart CT (2009) *The End of Materialism*: How evidence of the paranormal is bringing science and spirit together. Noetic Books, Institute of Noetic Sciences. New Harbinger Publications, Inc. Oakland, CA **Spirituality - quality science**

156 Unterwald EM (2008) Naltrexone in the treatment of alcohol dependence. J Addiction Medicine 2 (3): 121-7

157 Van der Kolk BA, Alexander C, McFarlane K, Weisaeth L (1996) Traumatic Stress: The Effects of Overwhelming Experience on Mind, Body, and Society. New York: Guilford Press

158 van Lommel P, interviewed by van Dusen M (2010) *Consciousness Beyond Life*: The science of the near-death experience. HarperCollins, NY "Psychiatry is supposed to promote mental health and instead it prevents it."

159 Warner CH, Bobo W, Warner C, Reid S, Rachal J (2006) Antidepressant Discontinuation Syndrome Am Fam Physician. 2006 Aug 1;74(3):449-456 online @ www.aafp.org/afp/2006/0801/p449.html

160 Weil AT: *From Chocolate to Morphine*: Everything You Need to Know About Mind-Altering Drugs. Mariner Books/ Houghton Mifflin Harcourt, NY, 2004

161 Whitaker R (2010) *Mad in America*: Bad Science, Bad Medicine, and the Enduring Mistreatment of the Mentally Ill Basic Books; 2nd Ed. **See also** his 13 p summary of key findings from his 2 books @ http://psychrights.org/litigation/WhitakerAffidavit.pdf

162 Whitaker R (2010) *Anatomy of an Epidemic*: Magic Bullets, Psychiatric Drugs, and the Astonishing Rise of Mental Illness in America. Basic Books, NY **See also** Bruce Levine interview http://www.alternet.org/health/146659/are_psychiatric_drugs_c ausing_the_astonishing_rise_of_mental_illness_in_america

163 Whitfield (Harris) B: *Spiritual Awakenings*: Insights of the Near-Death Experience and Other Doorways to Our Soul. Health Communications, Deerfield Beach, FL 1995

164 Whitfield CL: *Healing the Child Within*: Discovery & Recovery for Adult Children of Dysfunctional Families. Health Communications, Deerfield Beach, FL, 1987

165 Whitfield CL: *A Gift to Myself*: A personal workbook and guide to Healing the Child Within. Health Communications, Deerfield Beach , FL , 1990 ... also translated & published in French

166 Whitfield CL: *Co-dependence* - Healing the Human Condition. The new paradigm for helping professionals and people in recovery. Health Communications, Deerfield Beach , FL 1991

167 Whitfield CL: *Boundaries and Relationships*: Knowing, Protecting and Enjoying the Self. Health Communications, Deerfield Beach , FL 1993 ... also translated and published in French and Spanish editions

168 Whitfield CL: *Memory and Abuse*: Remembering and Healing the Effects of Trauma. Health Communications, Deerfield Beach , FL , 1995

169 Whitfield CL: Adverse childhood experience and trauma (editorial). American Journal of Preventive Medicine, 14(4):361-364, May 1998

170 Whitfield CL: Internal verification and corroboration of traumatic memories. Journal of Child Sexual Abuse 6(3):99-122,1997

171 Whitfield CL (1998). Internal evidence and corroboration of traumatic memories of child sexual abuse with addictive disorders. Sexual Addiction & Compulsivity 5:269–292

172 Whitfield CL, Silberg J, Fink P (eds): *Misinformation Concerning Child Sexual Abuse and Adult Survivors*. Haworth Press NY 2002

173 Whitfield CL (2003) *The Truth about Depression*: Choices for Healing. Health Communications, Deerfield Beach, FL
... also translated and published in Portuguese edition

174 Whitfield CL (2004a) *The Truth about Mental Illness*: Choices for healing. Health Communications, Deerfield Beach, FL

175 Whitfield CL (2004b) *My Recovery*: A personal plan for healing. Health Communications, Deerfield Beach, FL

176 Whitfield CL, Whitfield BH, Park R, Prevett J: *The Power of Humility* (2006) Choosing Peace over Conflict in Relationships. Health Communications, Deerfield Beach, FL,

177 Whitfield CL (2010) *Choosing God*: A Bird's-Eye-View of A Course in Miracles. Muse House Press, Atlanta

178 Whitfield CL (2010) *Teachers of God*: Further reflections on A Course in Miracles. Muse House Press, Atlanta, 2010

179 Whitfield CL (2010) Psychiatric Drugs as Agents of Trauma. Int J of Risk and Safety in Medicine 22:1-3 *Last issue 2010*

180 Wittmann L, Schredl M, Kramer M.2007 Dreaming in posttraumatic stress disorder: A critical review of phenomenology, psychophysiology and treatment. Psychother Psychosom. 76(1):25-39

181 Wood BL (1987). *Children of Alcoholism*: The Struggle for Self and Intimacy in Adult life. University Press, NY

182 Yahuda R, ed (1998) *Psychological Trauma*. American Psychiatric Press, Washington, DC

183 Young AH, Currie A (1997). Physicians' knowledge of antidepressant withdrawal effects: a survey. J Clin Psychiatry 58 Suppl 7: 28–30

184 Young A, Haddad P (2000) Discontinuation symptoms and psychotropic drugs. Lancet; 355:1184

185 Zur O, Nordmarken N (2007). *DSM*: Diagnosing for Money and Power: Summary of the Critique of the DSM. Online publication by Zur Institute. Retrieved 23 Aug 2010@ www.zurinstitute.com/dsmcritique.html. *They summarized*: The *DSM* is more a **political** document than a scientific one. Decisions regarding inclusion or exclusion of disorders are made by majority vote rather than by indisputable scientific data.

Added after above reference numbers were set

186 Breggin PR (2006) Intoxication Anosognosia: The Spellbinding Effect of Psychiatric Drugs. *Ethical Human Psychology and Psychiatry*, 8, 201-215

187 Hardman JG, Limbird LE (eds.) Goodman and Gilman's *The Pharmacologic Basis of Therapeutics* 9th ed., McGraw Hill, NY

188 Whitfield CL (in process for 2011) *Wisdom to Know the Difference*: Core Issues in relationships, recovery and life. Muse House Press, Atlanta

189 The Medicated Child; and Medicating Kids. 2 PBS documentaries, WGBH Boston Frontline

190 Guyol G (2010) *Who's Crazy Here*? Steps to recovery without drugs for ADD/ADHD, Addiction & Eating disorders, Anxiety & PTSD, Depression, Bipolar Disorder, Schizophrenia, Autism. Ajoite Publishing, CT

191 Silverman E (2010) In his blogs on http://www.pharmalot.com/

192 Emotional Freedom Technique @ http://eft.mercola.com/

193 Caplan PJ (1995). *They Say You're Crazy*: How the World's Most Powerful Psychiatrists Decide Who's Normal. Addison-Wesley, NY

194 Saisan J, de Benedictis J, Barston S, Segal R (2008) Sleeping Well; What You Need To Know: Sleep Requirements, Needs, Cycles and Stages. Retrieved May 30, 2009, from http://www.helpguide.org/life/sleeping.htm

195 Valenstein E (1998) *Blaming the Brain*: The Truth About Drugs and Mental Health, Free Press

Charles L. Whitfield, M.D.

196 Spiellmans GI (2009) The promotion of olanzapine [Zyprexa] in primary care: An examination of internal industry documents. Social Science & Medicine 69:14-20 **Another telling indictment of corruption in BigPharma**

197 Brodhagen A, Wise D (2008) Optimism as a mediator between the experience of child abuse, other traumatic events, and distress. J Family Violence 23:403-11

198 Kauffman JM (2009) Selective serotonin reuptake inhibitor (SSRI) drugs: More risks than benefits J Amer Physic & Surgeons 14 1:7-12

199 Tracy AB (1994/2001) *Prozac*: Panacea or Pandora? Cassia publications

200 Middleton H (2008) Whither DSM and ICD, Chapter 5? Mental Health Review Journal 13:4-15

About The Author

Charles L. Whitfield, M.D. is a physician, therapist and researcher with over 30 years of experience working with patients who have had childhood trauma, addiction and PTSD.

He is the best-selling author of *"Healing the Child Within," "Memory and Abuse," "The Power of Humility,"* and others.

He has written extensively on topics including the medical misrepresentation of diseases and the toxic drugs that the drug industry makes and indiscriminately sells through partially knowing clinicians to the unknowing public at high profit.

Two companion books on these topics are **The Truth About Depression** and **The Truth About Mental Illness**, in which he describes what are erroneously labeled "Mental Illnesses" and suggests safer, proven, more effective ways to heal these frequently painful conditions.

INDEX

Pain killer drugs, (*see Opiates*)
parents, 15, 17, 19, 26, 29, 30, 34-6, 39, 45, 49, 71-2, 82, 103, 114-7, 126, 132
passion flower extract, 149
patience, 18, 80, 139, 148, 160, 172
Perfectionism, 33
personal power, 39
personal recovery plan, 14, 173
Peter Breggin, v, vi, 68, 81, 86, 90, 114, 141-2, 145, 148, 183-4, 210-11, 215, 221, 223
pharmacists, 68
Phencyclidine (PCP), 67
Phenytoin (Dilantin), 65-6, 89
physical abuse, 23
physicians, 5-6, 12-14, 21, 56, 63, 66, 68, 73, 78-9, 108, 110-11, 114, 129, 130-2, 138, 140, 145, 149
Post-traumatic stress disorder (*see PTSD*)
Prison inmates, 116, 125
psychedelic, 67
Psychiatric Advanced Directive (PAD), 124-5
psychiatric symptoms, 58, 71, 94, 182-3, 215
psychological or emotional abuse, 23, 35
psychologists, 56
psychosis, 2, 16, 19, 47, 52, 57, 72, 74, 85, 93-5, 100, 117, 124, 192-3, 200, 202, 205ff
psychotherapy, 5, 6, 53-4, 63, 72-4, 79, 99, 116, 140, 163, 186
PTSD (*Post-Traumatic Stress Disorder*), 2-3, 15, 18, 20, 42, 43ff, 56-8, 61-5, 74, 76, 79, 81-2, 95-6, 107, 112, 115, 117, 123-4, 139, 144, 147-8, 155, 160-1, 171-3, 186-7, 189, 192-3, 198, 202-3, 213-4, 220

Quality multi vitamins, 148
quality of life, 5, 56, 67, 75, 84, 109, 116, 126, 178, 186, 206

Rage, 33, 52, 199
Real Self, (*see also True Self*) 15
Recovery, i-ii, xii, 1, 3-6, 14, 18-21, 30-1, 37, 39, 41-2, 52, 54-7, 60-5, 75,80-1, 89, 100-1, 109, 111, 113, 132, 138, 140, 144, 148, 159-60, 166-78, 180-4, 203, 206, 213, 220
relationship problems, 1, 6, 51, 55, 71-3, 76
REM (dream) sleep, 189
repeated childhood trauma, 9, 13, 23, 32, 36-7, 42, 72, 75, 98, 111
Resentment, 33
Restless leg syndrome, 186, 190
re-traumatization, 49
revictimization, 49
Richard Tranter, 69
risk/benefit ratio, 127
Risperdal (Risperidone), 85-6, 118, 136, 153
Ritalin (*see also methylphenidate*), 67, 70, 76, 193
Ritalin versus placebo, 103
Roland Summit, 48

Schizophrenia, 2, 86, 99-100, 161, 219
secret, 36, 129-30
Serenity Prayer, 112

More Titles by Charles and Barbara Whitfield

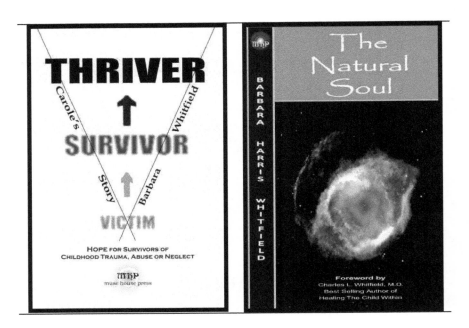

Available on Amazon.com and
Fine Booksellers Everywhere
by Muse House Press

More by Charles Whitfield

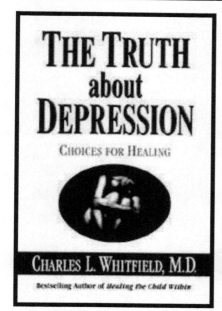

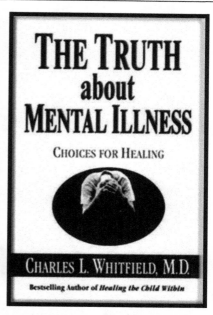

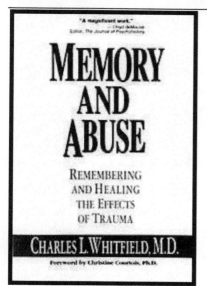

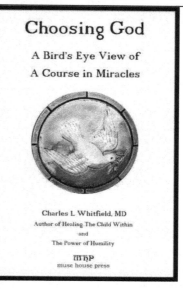

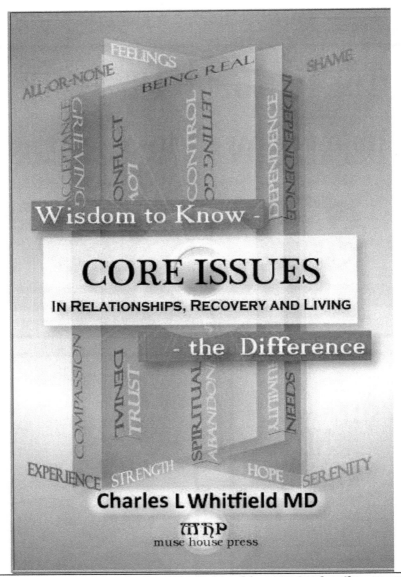

Wisdom to Know -

CORE ISSUES
IN RELATIONSHIPS, RECOVERY AND LIVING

- the Difference

Charles L Whitfield MD

ꟽꞪꝒ
muse house press

In this powerful book, Dr. Whitfield addresses in detail common Core Issues in relationships, recovery and life —how they come about and choices and solutions to use them to your advantage, heal and experience peace. He draws on over 35 years of experience assisting people to learn to identify and handle each Core Issue.

Charles L. Whitfield, M.D.